Roberta Zarpelão
Milva Maria F. de Martino

Quality of life and accidents among construction workers

Roberta Zarpelão
Milva Maria F. de Martino

Quality of life and accidents among construction workers

Psychosocial Aspects, Quality of Life and Sleep among injured and healthy outsourced workers

ScienciaScripts

Imprint

Cover image: www.ingimage.com

This book is a translation from the original published under ISBN 978-3-330-76713-3.

Publisher:
Sciencia Scripts
is a trademark of
Dodo Books Indian Ocean Ltd. and OmniScriptum S.R.L publishing group

120 High Road, East Finchley, London, N2 9ED, United Kingdom
Str. Armeneasca 28/1, office 1, Chisinau MD-2012, Republic of Moldova, Europe
Managing Directors: Ieva Konstantinova, Victoria Ursu
info@omniscriptum.com

Printed at: see last page
ISBN: 978-620-8-55109-4

The premise of this work is to assess the prevalence of accidents at work and compare quality of life, sleep patterns and psychosocial aspects between healthy and injured outsourced construction workers. The construction industry accounts for 10% of GDP and has peculiar characteristics, such as a low level of education, high rates of accidents at work, including fatal accidents, as well as a much-discussed component today, which is the precariousness of work through outsourced contracts. The topics discussed below are of current relevance, with up-to-date theoretical references, as they present instruments that allow the assessment of quality of life using the Whoqol-bref instrument, the Munich questionnaire that allows the assessment of employees' sleep patterns and the use of the Demand Control Support Questionnaire (DCSQ) model, which has been used to measure the work environment and its repercussions on various groups of workers, including construction workers.

DEDICATORY

I dedicate this book, which is yet another longed-for achievement in my life, to the construction workers, people of extreme competence with whom I have worked for seven years who, through their efforts, contribute to the development of the country

If there is no fruit, the beauty of the flowers is worth it
If there are no flowers
The shade of the leaves was worth it
If there are no leaves
The intention of the seeds was worth it (Heinfel

SUMMARY

Foreword

The basic theme of this book, which is a product of the PhD thesis developed by the authors in the Postgraduate Nursing Programme at the Federal University of São Paulo in 2015, is construction workers, work accidents and quality of life intertwined.

In this century's scenario, many peculiarities surround this professional category, and their difficulties at work and in life deserve to be studied in the search for solutions. With this study, the authors have managed to penetrate this group, showing results that are sometimes surprising and sometimes alarming.

It's always a pleasure to see the results of research and the full development of a young researcher. Having experienced Roberta reaching all the stages in our Programme, I can only congratulate her on this work, which I had the opportunity to read while it was still under construction.

Her advisor Prof Dr Milva Maria Figueiredo de Martino also deserves recognition for her constant support, guidance and partnership, which were fundamental in enabling this research to produce relevant results.

It's worth reading and getting involved with the bibliographical review that begins the book and which was designed to allow the reader to follow the course of the study. The description of the research, the method, the instruments used and the results obtained are a relevant source of learning and a reference for studies on this subject.

Congratulations to the authors!

And happy reading to all!
Prof Dr Isabel Cristina Kowal Olm Cunha
Associate Professor, Postgraduate Nursing Programme, UNIFESP

PRESENTATION

The interest in researching living and working conditions and the consequences of accidents at work for the health of construction workers stems from the concern that the influence and conditions of this specific environment have on the lives of these workers.

In this context, the main objective of this study is to compare the variables of QoL, sleep and control demand between the groups of healthy and injured construction workers.

The specific objectives are to identify the quality of life and sleep in the groups of healthy and injured individuals; to compare the groups of injured and healthy workers with regard to psychosocial aspects (control demand); to correlate the characteristics relating to sleep in the groups of healthy and injured individuals.

The main hypothesis of this study is that injured construction workers have worse QoL scores, demand control and less sleep than healthy workers.

Chapter 1 of this book will cover work in the construction industry, work in the construction industry; accidents at work; demand control; quality of life and the characteristics of the sleep-wake cycle.

Chapter 2 will deal with the demand for control at work; work and accidents; sleep disorders and quality of life at work in the construction industry.

Chapter 3 will deal with general considerations; hypotheses; objectives; sample; instrument; procedures; statistical analysis; results; discussion and conclusion.

Roberta Zaninelli do Nascimento
Milva Maria Figueiredo de Martino

CHAPTER 1

Work in the construction industry, its peculiarities and demands

Important events have occurred in human history, each in its own time, such as the Taylor-Fordist accumulation crisis (1965-1975), characterised by important facts such as the radicalisation and hardening of workers' union movements; the mismatch between capital appreciation and productivity growth; the shock of rising oil prices; the rise in interest rates in the early 1970s; and the reduction in investment, which had an impact on employment and income rates. It was in this context that a process of productive restructuring took hold, bringing about institutional changes in production and labour relations, as well as in the role of national states. On the whole, the changes in the production scenario in Western capitalist societies are accompanied by the following characteristics: a reduction in the role of the state; government policies to increase the value of financial capital; more flexible labour contracts; a growing increase in unemployment rates and social exclusion; and a low and unstable expansion of wealth for society as a whole (Ferreira et al., 2009; Rocha et al., 2014).

The acceleration of changes in the world of work, especially the fast and intense pace of technological innovations in the information society; the increase in knowledge content added to production; the shortening of the life cycle of products, production processes changing at high speed and the so-called "knowledge industries" growing and demanding more qualified professionals with skills that have to be constantly updated (Ferreira et al., 2009).

According to Ferreira et al. (2009), "the winds of change", driven by globalisation, are seeking to transform institutions in order to make them more efficient and with a reduced workforce. Thus, a change is taking place in the landscape of traditional professions, requiring flexible specialisation (adding new tasks), functional flexibility (rotation of activities, multi-skilling) and polytechnics (complex tasks, creative skills). The "new worker" is expected to develop the skills to handle new technological tools, deal with less structured problems, relate socially (communication, negotiation, conflict resolution), work in teams and take on new responsibilities to work in environments with greater uncertainty and poorly defined roles (Ferreira et al., 2009).

In recent decades, changes in the work environment have triggered changes in the relationship between work, stress and its repercussions, as well as issues such as productivity, accidents at work, absenteeism and growing statistics related to physical and psychological symptoms among workers in certain professional categories. These include teachers, health professionals and lorry drivers, given the many stressful circumstances in their daily working lives (Magnano et al., 2010).

Research shows that work has paradoxical consequences for the physical and psychological integrity of individuals. If, on the one hand, it is seen as a productive activity, seen as the worker's identity, with a fundamental role that guarantees their health; on the other hand, when it takes on the meaning of something painful, that is carried out in precarious conditions and that does not offer opportunities for professional development, it can contribute to workers becoming ill, as a result of compulsion to work (workaholic), as well as non-work and unemployment (Santos et al., 2010; Choi, Kang, 2010).

Studies show that the association between job insecurity and workers' health, which generates psychological distress, some physical symptoms and low esteem, is mentioned by some authors in their articles, reporting that working conditions, organisational and social structures and individual characteristics may be related, thus increasing the risk of accidents at work (Ghisi et al., 2013; Virtanen et al., 2013).

Because of its peculiar characteristics, the possibility of a worker having an accident, falling ill or even dying is significant. It's important to check the conditions under which workers are working in this segment of the economy, as well as the knowledge about health risk prevention adopted in people management, which makes them perform their duties with motivation and satisfaction, feeling valued and satisfied as human beings, since health is directly related to quality of life (QoL) (Ferraz, Aquino, 2014).

According to Dataprev, in 2012 there were 423,935 typical accidents at work (TA) in Brazil, and 159,047 cases in the south-east of the country (Brasil, 2012).

The construction industry is a sector of recognised importance due to its purpose and scope, which is contradictorily marked by the constant coexistence with risky situations, proven by the high number of accidents at work, including disabling and fatal ones; it is also marked by incipient preventive actions, in which these characteristics can cause aggravations to workers' health, with repercussions on their QoL, as well as their sleep.

The history of the world allows us to say that the construction industry has always existed to meet the basic and immediate needs of man, without any concern for health and safety at first (Corrêa, 2009).

Construction is an economic activity that makes a major contribution to any country's gross domestic product, with its own peculiar characteristics and significant effects on employment. With more than 11 million workers, the construction industry represents one of the largest industries in the United States of America and accounts for 5% of the Gross Domestic Product in Brazil (Ferraz, Aquino, 2014; Azevedo et al., 2011; Jacobsen et al., 2013).

It has a large number of workers associated with the construction of buildings and large structures, such as hydroelectric power stations, bridges, among others. The European view of motorway construction has divided construction workers into two categories: workers exposed to hazardous potential and office workers (Lykouras et al., 2014; Ferraz, Aquino, 2014).

Civil construction is one of the most important activities in the country and accounts for approximately 3.5 million jobs in Brazil, which corresponds to 6% of the total. Most of these workers come from the Northeast region, with low levels of education, where some groups of workers, including those in the textile industry and electricity companies, have between 1 and 8 years of schooling and limited socioeconomic conditions (Ferraz, Aquino, 2014; Serkalem et al., 2014; Kalte et al., 2014; Galdino et al., 2012).

On the other hand, workers in electricity companies and construction in general are represented by male workers (Kalte et al., 2014; Galdino et al., 2012). However, in informal working conditions, according to Sotelo-Suárez et al. (2012) in Bogotá, Colombia, the percentage is predominantly female, which was not found in this study.

The term "outsourcing" was coined by Aldo Sani in the early 1970s. The word "outsourcing" is a neologism used exclusively in Brazil; in other countries, it is taken to mean the relationship between two companies, i.e. it is always the translation of the word subcontracting: in French, soustraitance; in Italian, sobcontrattazione; in Spanish, subcontratación; in English, outsourcing; in Portugal, subcontratação (Marcelino, Cavalcante, 2012).

According to the Annual Social Information Report - RAIS (2013), established by Decree 76.900 of 23/12/75, the distribution of outsourced workers in Brazil in 2013 was 26.80%. Table 1 shows outsourcing in Brazil in 2013 - (26.80%).

In a large oil industry, the ratio between the number of outsourced workers in 1995 was approximately 46,000 to 29,000, respectively. In 2013, there were 62,000 own workers and 320,000 outsourced workers, representing a ratio of 5 outsourced workers for every own worker (Central Única dos Trabalhadores, 2014).

Table 1. Distribution of workers in typically outsourced and typically contracted sectors, S.P. 2013

Sectors	**Number of Workers**	**2013**
Typical contracting sectors	34.748.421 73,2	73,20
Typically outsourced sectors	127.005.46,00	26,80
Total	47.448.967 100,00	100,00

Source: Ministry of Labour and Employment (BR) (2013).

Accidents at work

Accidents at work are considered a serious public health problem in Brazil and worldwide (Bordoni et al., 2016). The World Health Organisation

Health (WHO) defines accidents at work as a public health problem and epidemic in developing countries (Moradinazar et al., 2013).

An accident at work (AT) is defined by the Ministry of Social Welfare and Assistance as one that occurs during the course of work or while travelling on company business, which causes bodily injury or functional disturbance; or which causes death, loss or reduction, permanent or temporary, of capacity for work (Brasil, 2013).

Accidents at work in industry are more frequent than in other sectors. In the United States, in 2010, construction had the highest number of fatal accidents; in Brazil, accidents at work represent the main health problem for workers, as well as being complex and multi-causal phenomena, which can reveal a dysfunction in management and work organisations (Prestes et al., 2012; Jacobsen et al., 2014; Almeida et al., 2014).

Statistics on accidents at work are published annually, but due to underreporting, these figures are not very reliable. In 1998, only 3.9% of accidents at work worldwide were recorded, according to the International Labour Organisation (ILO), and there were around 270 million accidents at work, with 350,000 deaths per year worldwide (Mehrdad et al., 2014; Abas et al., 2013; Lacerda et al., 2014).

According to the International Labour Organisation, one in 10 workers is involved in personal injuries every year, and 5% of working days are lost. In studies carried out in the United States of America (USA), the cost of accidents at work was $177,200,000,000, with 35 million working days wasted annually (Moradinazar et al., 2013).

It is estimated that in 2009, according to Eurostat, around 2.8 million accidents occurred in the European Union (Ghisi et al., 2013). According to Cofindustria - Italy, in 2011 there was a 10.9 per cent drop in accidents in the construction sector compared to previous years (Tomei et al., 2015).

According to a study carried out in Peru, between 2011 and 2014 there was a decrease in fatal and non-fatal accidents at work among construction workers , although the city of Lima is considered to have the highest number of non-fatal accidents (Mejia et al., 2015).

It was only in the 20th century that possible occupational diseases and their relationship with copper were related in Chile, concatenating that the work environment and the conditions to which the worker is exposed can generate diseases among them silicosis in the case of exposure to copper and or accidents at work (Almont et al., 2016).

Another example might be mining, which is known to be an intrinsically dangerous occupation worldwide. Workers in underground mines are exposed to various risks, including openings, improper ventilation, heat and humidity, noise and vibration, poor lighting, dust in the air, as well as harmful gases and slippery floors that can cause additional stress on workers (Bhattacherejje, Kuna, 2016).

The current development of the electric power industry in Poland, especially in the field of renewable energy sources, including wind power, brings the need to introduce new labour environment legislation (Piotrowiski et al., 2016)

And today, construction workers globally face disproportionate threats to their health and well-being, constituted by the nature of the work they do (Dutta, 2017).

In India, the construction industry is the second largest employer compared to agriculture. The construction sector is manual, heavy and complex, with the highest incidence of fatalities and occupational diseases, as well as long periods of sick leave for these reasons (Kim, Minm Jung, 2017;Yi,Chan , 2016; Kanchana , Sivaprakash , Sebastian J, 2015).

Global estimates from the International Labour Organization (ILO), reported more than 60.000 deaths a year and that these deaths occurred in the construction sector, according to the US Bureau of Labour Statistics, which reported that construction sites had the highest number of fatal injuries, with 899 fatal injuries in 2014; while in the United Kingdom there were 217 fatalities in 2010, in Hong Kong the number of accidents in the construction sector was 20 with 3467 accidents in the same year, in Korea between 2001 and 2015 there were 225 accidents, with 173 deaths and the most serious refers to the construction of a tunnel with approximately 56 accidents with 30 deaths and in Spain this rate is even higher with 350 deaths per year, in Brazil in the year 2010 there were 2800 fatal accidents with invaluable losses in addition to the financial ones (Yi, Chan, 2017; Bordoni et al., 2016).

The fishing industry is one of the most dangerous in the world, while the construction industry is responsible for a large part of the gross domestic product and is also considered one of the most dangerous in the world. In the construction industry there are various functions that workers carry out throughout the day, and the result is a high incidence of accidents at work, up to even deaths caused by heat-related stress (Chauvin et al., 2017; Suarez et al., 2017).

Various factors contribute to occupational injuries and most research has focused on identifying factors that contribute to the workplace. Known risk factors such as younger age group, male gender and low education, as well as long working hours per day, insecurity and with globalisation the forms of employment contract, such as casual workers, temporary and "floating" contracts, self-employment, "home office", domestic work, tele-service among others may appear as factors that increase the incidence of occupational accidents (Dutta, 2017; Alali et al., 2016).

In addition to the factors mentioned above that make up the precarious work often carried out by migrants, there is a lack of access to resources such as insurance, health care and others, poor worker protection policies with little protection for migrants and an almost always unskilled workforce (Dutta, 2017). These employment arrangements are characterised by lower income, poor job security, knowledge of workplace risks and health risks, in which case women are more susceptible (Alali et al., 2016).

In 2010, 14% of workers in Europe were in temporary work, 65% in Kosovo and 1% in Romania (Alali et al., 2016). Studies carried out in India, Korea and Italy found that the occurrence of accidents at work was higher among outsourced workers who were not regulated by law compared to workers who were covered by legislation among outsourced workers, while other studies carried out in Finland and Spain found contradictory results when it came to accidents at work (Alali et al., 2016).

According to a study by Alali (2016), low schooling can be a factor in the occurrence of accidents at work, and in this same study temporary workers did not have a higher injury rate than permanent workers.

Despite the downward trend in accidents at work in developed countries, globalisation has contributed to an increase in accidents at work in developing countries (Mehrdad et al., 2014; Abas et al., 2013).

OAs harm the country's productivity and economy, as workers can be absent from their work for a period of two to three days, with an estimated cost of approximately 268 million in 2001, as well as great suffering, with psychological and family repercussions that are difficult to measure (Mehrdad et al., 2014; Socias et al., 2014; Abas et al., 2013; Lacerda et al., 2014). It is estimated that accidents at work can account for around 10% of the gross domestic product (GDP) in economic and social costs (Vilela et al., 2012).

In Brazil, around 717,900 accidents at work were registered with the National Social Security Institute (INSS) in 2013. Of the total number of accidents recorded with a Communication of Accident at Work - CAT, typical accidents accounted for 77.32%, commuting accidents for 19.96% and occupational diseases for 2.72%. Males accounted for 73.01% and females for 26.99% of typical accidents; 62.21% and 37.79% of commuting accidents; and 58.38% and 41.62% of occupational diseases. In typical and commuting accidents, the age group with the highest incidence of accidents was people aged 20 to 29, with 34.11 per cent and 37.50 per cent respectively of all accidents recorded. In the case of occupational diseases, the age group with the highest incidence was between 30 and 39 years old, with 33.52% of all accidents recorded (Brasil, 2013).

Countries differ in terms of which industry is considered the most dangerous. In the United States, commercial fishing is one of the most dangerous professions, representing an annual mortality rate of 129 deaths per 100,000 fishermen in 2008, while the average occupation by lethality for all other North American workers is 4/100,000 (Abas et al., 2013).

The mining, agricultural and construction industries accounted for the highest incidence of fatalities in the Republic of Korea, 34/100,000, and the construction sector is considered the most dangerous (Abas et al., 2013).

In Taiwan in 2004, the Labour Relations Board noted that falls were the main cause of work-related deaths and were higher among men compared to women (men, 7.4 per 100,000, women, 0.9 per 100,000). Different statistics were found in Malaysia, where the agricultural sector had the highest incidence, with 24.1/1000, followed by the subcategories of the wood products manufacturing sector, with 22.1/1000 (Abas et al., 2013).

In 2013, the subgroups of the Brazilian Occupation Code (CBO) with the highest number of typical accidents were 'Transversal function workers' and 'Service workers', with 14.49 per cent and 15.09 per cent, respectively (Brazil, 2013).

By sector of economic activity, the Agriculture and livestock sector accounted for 3.47% of all accidents registered with a CAT; the Industry sector accounted for 45.48% and the Services sector 51.05%, excluding data on ignored activities. With regard to typical accidents, the sub-sectors with the largest share of accidents were Trade and Repair of Motor Vehicles, with 12.61 per cent, and Health and Social Services, with 12.08 per cent of the total (Brazil, 2013).

In 2013, of the 50 ICD (International Classification of Diseases) codes with the highest incidence in accidents at work, the ones with the highest participation were injuries to the wrist and hand (S61), fractures of the wrist or hand (S62) and superficial trauma to the wrist and hand (S60), with 9.59%, 6.91% and 4.84% of the total, respectively (Ministry of Social Security, 2013).

The parts of the body with the highest incidence of typical accidents were the fingers, the hand (except the wrist or fingers) and the foot (except the toes), with 29.93 per cent, 8.60 per cent and 7.67 per cent respectively (Ministry of Social Security, 2013).

In 2013, the number of work-related accidents compiled was approximately 737,400, which was an increase of 0.40 per cent compared to 2012. Medical care fell by 0.13 per cent and fatalities increased by 1.05 per cent compared to 2012. Temporary disabilities increased by 0.87 per cent and permanent disabilities fell by 12.96 per cent. The main consequences of accidents at work were temporary disabilities of less than 15 days and more than 15 days, which accounted for 46.04% and 36.79% of the total, respectively (Brazil, 2013).

Even today, a reductionist and biased view prevails that accidents have one or a few causes stemming from human error, unsafe acts, behaviour, among others associated with non-compliance with safety norms and standards; or technical and material failures, an approach inherited from classical disciplines such as Occupational Hygiene, which is insufficient to explain the causes of accidents and their harmfulness, limiting surveillance and prevention actions and leaving the determinants of these events untouched (Vilela et al., 2012).

Prevention can arise from actions and strategies that are articulated and worked on in groups, in order to analyse and intervene in the factors that determine and result from the circumstances of health problems related to work processes (Vilela et al., 2012).

Accidents can be influenced by aspects of the immediate work situation such as: the machinery, the task, the technical or material environment; but also by working relationships, organisational culture, as well as fatigue (Patterson et al., 2015; Vilela et al., 2012). The work environment is a reservoir of various stressors, both physical and psychological (Tomei et al., 2015).

With the changes taking place in the world, there is a need to understand the risk factors for accidents at work today (Basnet et al., 2010).

Sleep changes

The systematic study of day and night shift work or rotating shifts has contributed to a better understanding of the consequences for workers' health (De Queirós, Lima, 2013).

Work has been present in man's relationship with nature since ancient times, in which human beings, through their own actions, drive, regulate and control their material exchange with nature, and it was through work that other human functions and behaviours developed (De Queirós, Lima, 2013).

It is in the sphere of social reproduction that new needs and possibilities are generated, which will give rise to new social relations, such relations being organised in the form of social complexes, social needs such as health can be defined according to the social classes to which they belong (De Queirós, Lima, 2013).

The changes that have taken place in the world of work have had a direct impact on workers' health, and the growing demand for new technologies, added to a complex set of organisational innovations, has interfered with working conditions and relationships (Mendes, De Martino, 2012).

The intensification of work is an element of the current phase of capitalism that involves the consumption of workers' physical and spiritual energies. These transformations have a direct impact on workers' health as a result of the work process needing to be reorganised to meet the characteristics of each profession (Mendes, De Martino, 2012). Shift work is not an invention of the industrial age, it has existed since the organisation of cities and states (Mendes, De Martino, 2012).

Day and night work, regardless of the form or location of the work activities, has existed for millennia, especially in strategic commercial locations. The structuring of work in shift systems in contemporary society is increasing the number of services that generally operate for periods of 12, 14 and 24 hours, so shift work has gradually increased in the last decade due to society's own demand for the services required, which makes night work or irregular hours increasingly frequent (Fujiki, 2013);

Many circadian rhythms are controlled by cells in the hypothalamic region, in the Suprachiasmatic Nucleus, also influenced by external synchronisers such as light and dark, feeding, among others, but they also persist without these environmental cues, which characterises them as endogenously generated rhythms (Mohebbi, Shateri , Seyed , 2012).

The disruption of both the internal and external temporal order can lead to health problems, often responsible for accidents, lack of interest, anxiety, irritability, loss of efficiency and stress, which have repercussions on workers' quality of life (Dorrian, et al., 2012, Guimarães LBM, Pessa BSLR, Biguelini 2012).

There are reliable indications that individual characteristics are important in coping with such disturbances. Thus, an ever-present question is to understand what strategies are involved in each individual's adaptation to the manipulation of external temporal schemes (Mohebbi, Shateri , Seyed , 2012).

People who work shifts or specifically night shifts often have poor sleep quality during the day. This is due to social conflicts and excessive daytime noise. This poor quality of sleep will lead to increased sleepiness during the working period, whether night or day, and sleep disorders have a high social cost (Dos Santos, De Martino, 2013).

The balance between the influences of the synchronisers and the internal temporal order can be disturbed by abrupt changes in working hours, trans-meridian flights or night work.

With increasing age, certain characteristics of biological rhythms change and are somewhat associated with tolerance to shift work. Some studies have shown that older people (55-60 years old) prefer to go to sleep earlier than they used to, i.e. they show a reduction in total sleep time (TST), so over the years people become more morning-orientated, which can make social and family life more difficult (Dorrian et al., 2012; Ljosa CH, Tyssen R, Lau B, 2012).

Knowing the characteristics of workers' mornings and afternoons can help define periods of better physical and mental performance, contributing to the prevention of health problems.

Although the function of sleep is not fully understood12, sleep is characterised by a reduction in response to stimuli, reversibility, continuous movement, stereotypical posture, specific to each species, individual duration and times for each species and has a restorative function, as well as interfering with mood, memory, attention, sensory registers, reasoning, in short, cognitive aspects that relate a person to their environment and determine the quality of their performance and health. 13

Scholars say that sleep is just as important for maintaining good health as eating well (Anacleto, 2013).

The circadian rhythm and homeostatic control are the major determinants of the sleep-wake cycle, although other behavioural parameters such as body temperature, hormone secretion, cardiopulmonary function, cognitive performance and mood also exhibit circadian rhythmicity (Araújo, Almondes, 2012).

It has been observed that two hours before waking up, people's core temperature tends to be at its lowest, gradually increasing due to the concentration of cortisol in the blood close to the moment they wake up. On the other hand, nocturnal sleep, guided by the absence of light, favours the release of growth hormone and prolactin, substances that are fundamental to vital functions. 18

Sleep is the rhythmic activity of human beings, and this rhythmicity of biological systems has developed over the course of evolution so that adaptation has occurred to changes in the environment with the physiology of organisms (Sridhar, Sanjana, 2016).

Some sleep disorders, including sleep apnoea, can cause nocturnal drowsiness and lack of concentration, leading to traffic accidents and are considered a public health problem; it's worth noting that identifying and treating snoring can reduce the number of occupational injuries, absenteeism, improved productivity, absenteeism, health and well-being of these professionals (Guimarães, Hermont, 2014).

Insomnia, which is a sleep disorder, can be linked to workplace injuries, as it decreases workers' safety behaviours and continues to have high human and economic costs (Kao, et al., 2016).

Characteristics of the Sleep-Wake Cycle

Due to the increase in industrialisation in society, working shifts or at night has become common practice, but it is known that sleep plays a fundamental role in people and has repercussions on work and daily life. Its absence or failure can result in daytime sleepiness, leading to economic and social impacts, becoming a risk factor for diseases such as metabolic syndrome, risks of accidents at work, as well as changes in the sleep-wake cycle, which cause damage to workers' QoL (Wagstaff, Segstad, 2011; Lykouras et al., 2014; Raja et al., 2015; Fossum et al., 2013; Fujiki, 2013; De Martino, 2009; Ferreira, De Martino, 2012).

Excessive physical effort and high work demands are considered risk indicators for sleep disorders (De Martino, 2009).

The sleep-wake cycle is directly influenced by night work, as well as various other circadian rhythms, and considering that individuals have daytime habits, their QoL can be altered (De Martino, 2009).

Shift work is defined as taking place between 19:00 and 06:00, so night work involves shift work and the vast majority work from 22:00 to 06:00 (Fossum et al., 2013).

Some factors can affect the quality and quantity of sleep: jet lag, other circadian factors (time of day), shift work and, among them, occupational stress, which is considered a possible risk factor for insomnia. The relationship between stress and sleep disorders is due to the high secretion of cortisol, which is one of the brain's endocrine regulators activated from the hypothalamus-pituitary gland axis, responsible for inducing sleep disorders, capable of generating occupational stress

(Khaleghipour et al., 2015; Johnson et al., 2014; De Martino, 2009).

In a recent survey carried out in an industry in Norway, Fossum et al. (2013) showed that 55 per cent of workers work shifts. The shift is characterised by 12 by 24 hours, considered longer and different when compared to workers who work in onshore oil units. While offshore workers work two weeks at sea and two weeks at home, most Norwegian shift workers spend two weeks at sea and four weeks offshore. Shift rotations are fixed, 14 consecutive (day) shifts 14D and or 14 (night) shifts 14 N, alternated with tours or swing changes, comprising one week of night shifts (usually the first one) and one week of day shifts within the same job, period (7N / 7D) 27). In addition, offshore workers work in isolation from family, friends and society. The period at sea involves a lot of working time, enclosed environments, as well as safety courses and strict medical standards to ensure that employees are physically and mentally fit to carry out their activities for hours at a time (Fossum et al., 2013).

The majority of TAs are avoidable and approximately 16-20% of all traffic accidents and 29-50% of deaths and serious injuries are related to the human condition and not to technical faults. Many studies show that excessive sleepiness or sleep deprivation has similar effects to high blood alcohol concentration and is related to accidents involving transport and other modalities, which impairs vigilance and reaction time, including flights and train operation, among Argentinian and Brazilian drivers and health professionals (Wagstaff, Segstad, 2011; Johnson et al., 2014; Herman et al., 2014).

Drivers and healthcare professionals are more vulnerable, because in addition to physical factors such as fatigue and circadian desynchronisation with detrimental effects on human performance, the potential effects of working hours, there are also unfavourable conditions such as decision-making, socio-economic pressures and long periods of activity without adequate rest (Wagstaff, Segstad, 2011; Herman et al., 2014).

In research carried out by Vegso et al. (2007) with workers in the aluminium industry in the United States, as part of the continuous analysis of safety and health, it was based on a crossover study with 1955 individuals and it was observed that the incidence of accidents at work is higher when the hours worked are > 50 hours, and the opposite occurs when the number of hours worked is <40 hours (Wagstaff, Segstad, 2011).

In studies carried out in Germany, the correlation between the occurrence of accidents and the time of starting work was analysed. The results showed a high number of accidents for people who started their shift at 06:00, 07:00 and 08:00. A small peak was recorded in people who started their shift at 22:00 - 24:00 hours (Wagstaff, Segstad, 2011). When the accident was related to the duration of work, this study showed that the risk of serious accidents is exponentially higher when it exceeds 9ª working hours and, in a particular situation, when the start time differs from the usual working hours. However, whether it is day or night in this study had no clear effect on the risk of accidents.

In a survey of construction workers in the United States of America, the data analysed using statistical regression methods showed that when workers work for more than eight hours a day, there are more accidents at work compared to those who work seven or eight hours a day (Wagstaff, Segstad, 2011). Another study carried out with night workers showed a relative risk of accidents at work compared to those working conventional hours (Wagstaff, Segstad, 2011).

CHAPTER 2

Working conditions, quality of life

The implications of work on workers' health are due to actual changes in the labour world (Cavedom, 2014).

Research into the repercussions of work on workers' health in the 1970s was one-dimensional, based mainly on the demands of the tasks or related to the demands versus the individual's abilities to cope with them, and the worker's control over the methodology was not part of the analysis of the processes that produce work-related stress (Griep et al., 2011).

At the end of the 1970s, Robert Karasek proposed a new two-dimensional research model that defines work-related stress as a consequence of the combination of high psychological demands and low job control, which describes the combination of described ability and decision-making power (Chungkham et al., 2013).

Psychological demand is related to the demands that workers face in carrying out their activities (time pressure, level of concentration, interruption of tasks and the need to wait for other workers) (Griep et al., 2011).

Worker control is related to two aspects: the use of skills (the degree to which work involves learning) and decision-making authority (ability to make decisions at work and influence management policy) (Griep et al., 2011).

The assessment of the psychosocial work environment is based on the combination of high and low levels of these two dimensions, which are configured into four specific work situations that suggest different health risks: high demand (high demand and low control) which are the most adverse reactions of psychological wear and tear; active work (high psychological demand and high control) which allows the worker to have a wide possibility of deciding how and when to carry out their tasks, as well as using their intellectual potential for this purpose; passive work (low psychological demand and low control) which produces a gradual atrophy of skills learning and low demand (combines low demand and high control) which is configured in a highly comfortable and ideal state of work (Schioler et al., 2015; Griep et al., 2011; Magnano et al., 2010a).

Occupational stress can be understood as the interaction between high psychological demands, less control in the work production process and less social support received from colleagues and bosses. This condition can have harmful consequences for the worker's physical or mental health, i.e. those who are faced with high psychological demands or pressures at work, combined with low control or low decision-making power, can be at serious risk of falling ill as a result of psychological distress (Griep et al., 2011).

The Demand-Control Model (DCM) seeks to explain the changes that take place in individuals subjected to stress at work, both on a physiological and psychological level, and has been pointed out as a possible integrative framework for studying the various elements of the work environment, in their interrelationships with workers' health (Griep et al., 2011).

The MDC model considered the interaction of two components that could favour job strain: psychological demands (pace and intensity of work) and control (autonomy and ability) for the worker to carry out their work, so activities that involved high psychological demands and low control favoured job strain, resulting in physical and psychological illness. The model later included a third dimension: the perception of social support (Griep et al., 2011).

The Demand Control Support Questionnaire (DCSQ) model defines different work stressors that are potentially harmful to health and offers explanations of the relationship between stressful work conditions and physical and psychological wellbeing, and thus the model suggests that job strain generates an imbalance between perceived psychosocial stressors, including high productivity and lack of control over one's work. Job strain was associated with unhealthy behaviours that favour weight gain, such as physical inactivity, In comparison with other European countries, on the one hand, Danish workers perceive the greatest control over their work and, on the other hand, they are among the countries with the greatest control over their work.

Work intensity, regardless of the shorter weekly working time (Gralle A, et al., 2017; Griep, Rotemberg, Landsbergis, Silva, 2011; Thielen, Nygaard, Andersen, Diderichsen, 2014).

The Demand Control Support Questionnaire (DCSQ) is based on the psychosocial characteristics of work, the psychological demand involved in carrying out occupational tasks and activities and the control exercised by workers over their own work and the social support they receive. These items are part of occupational health and have been addressed more frequently through a questionnaire initially proposed by Karasek in a broad version and summarised by Theorell et al. (2001).

Studies carried out mainly in European countries, Asia and the United States of America have shown evidence of a positive association between psychosocial aspects of work (high psychological demand and low control) and different outcomes, such as minor psychiatric problems, diseases of the digestive system, musculoskeletal disorders, cardiovascular diseases, among others (Chungkham et al., 2013; Griep et al., 2011).

There has been an expansion of MDC in other countries, such as those in Latin America, in the last decade, as well as an increase in scientific productions in the period from 1979 to 2010 (Griep et al., 2011), but still few mention and analyse the issue of accidents at work due to the psychological demand and control in the work process (Brito, 2007), which can be considered a contributing factor in altering workers' QoL.

New needs in labour relations are emerging in a scenario of major transformations, as well as major and complex problems of all kinds affecting workers (Tabeleão, Tomasi, Neves, 2011, Knardahl et al., 2014; Mascarenhas et al., 2014).

The workplace presents individuals with a variety of challenges from work tasks and social interactions. Work also provides opportunities for positive fulfilment, achievement and friendship (Teles et al., 2014).

Occupation is still an important determinant in general and its overall positive or negative impact and effect on well-being results from the interaction between individual characteristics, the latter being made up of biomechanical, psychosocial and sociological axes (Lourenço et al., 2015).

For many, work is a social activity, a crucial source of feedback and can be a central component of personal identity, thus generating or not generating health and quality of life. Thus, working conditions can represent a particularly salient influence on emotions, self-esteem, and identity. Although employment is usually assumed to promote health, the net effect on mental health depends on the psychosocial quality of the job (WHO, 1995; Tabeleão, Tomasi, Neves, 2011, Knardahl et al., 2014).

Companies that care about the well-being and quality of life of their employees can improve working conditions and reduce conflicts, as well as absenteeism, *turnover* and better results (Giorgi, Dubin, Prerez, 2016).

Employee well-being has received a large amount of research interest in recent years, as it reflects on potential returns, increased productivity and worker loyalty (Giorgi, Dubin, Prerez, 2016; Soh et al., 2016).

The interaction of different conditions leads to working environments that are more or less favourable to health (Griep, Rotemberg, Landsbergis, 2011).

Previous studies indicate that psychological, social and organisational factors at work contribute to health, motivation, absence from work and functional capacity (Knardahl et al., 2014).High and increasing levels of mental morbidity, especially depression, and work demands may be the causes (Thielen, Nygaard, Andersen, Didrechsen, 2014; Gralle et al., 2017).

When it comes to working conditions, Danish workers have high job mobility due to low job protection, and high turnover, i.e. these workers change jobs 40 per cent more often than the rest of the European Union (Thielen, Nygaard, Andersen, Didrechsen, 2014).

The economic flows and productivity-driven pressures placed on construction workers can contribute to the onset of illness (Dutta, 2017).

Quality of Life

Quality of life can be defined as an individual's perception of their position in life, in the culture and value system in which they live, and in relation to their expectations, standards and concerns (Campos et al., 2014).

Historically, the only relevant aspects for determining QoL were material, but over time this concept has evolved, with personal satisfaction and fulfilment, quality of relationships, leisure options, access to cultural events, perception of general well-being, among others, being valued (Brum et al., 2012).

There are various concepts of QoL, but it is a fact that meeting basic needs - food, housing, education and work - form a fundamental component in assessing QoL. The subject has become so broad that QoL directly involves well-being, happiness, dreams, dignity, work and citizenship.

Quality of life is defined by the World Health Organisation (WHO) as a person's understanding of their position in life in terms of culture and values, considering their goals, expectations, standards and perceptions, and Quality of Life at Work can also be understood as a balance or reconciliation between work and other spheres of life (Marconato, Monteiro 2015, Padilha, 2009).

Some authors refer to two conceptions of QoL: lifestyles and living conditions. The first relates to the way people act, their behaviour, their life; the second relates to economic and demographic aspects. Thus, we can say that QoL at work is very much a result of the condition of life at work, in terms of economic and emotional aspects, as well as spirituality (Brum et al., 2012; Cavedon, 2014).

QoL is thinking along the lines of increasing life expectancy, with the key element being, in addition to meeting basic needs, improving lifestyle by acquiring healthy habits, taking part in physical activity, having stable, lasting relationships, a healthy diet, etc., because only in this way will we have healthy adults today and elderly people tomorrow.

The subject of QoL is broad and directly involves well-being, happiness, dreams, dignity, work and citizenship (Brum et al., 2012). Good QoL is the result of a complex interaction between factors such as psychological state, expectations, beliefs, values, social relationships and the environment (Ogata, Simurro, 2009).

It is clear that it is not feasible to restrict health and illness issues to the organisational scenario, since the health/disease binomial is linked to the different social actors and depends on the way people live, their QoL and their access to goods and services (Cavedon, 2014).

At the end of the 20th century, changes in organisations and the nature of work underwent a number of modifications, above all in order to meet the requirements of current legislation and competitiveness. Companies have increasingly invested in working conditions and the QoL and well-being of workers, with the aim of reducing the harmful effects that the organisational and work context can have on these individuals (Silva, Ferreira, 2013).

Work is one of the means of ensuring the satisfaction of personal needs and becomes a determining factor in QoL. Workers must be guaranteed certain rights, such as: a good working environment, good physical, emotional and material conditions to perform satisfactorily (Almeida et al., 2014).

QoL has been defined as the individual's subjective perception of their satisfaction at work, often through definitions that emphasise characteristics of the workplace, the organisational environment and the effects of certain conditions in the environment and the organisation on the individual's health and well-being, such as working conditions, equipment and the physical environment, among others (Silva, Ferreira, 2013).

Well-being at work consists of the results of the individual's assessment of the conditions at work, including cognitive, affective, motivational, psychosomatic and behavioural components. As such, it can stem from individuals' perception of the satisfaction of their needs and desires based on organisational performance, manifesting itself through feelings and gratification (Silva, Ferreira, 2013).

QoL should be seen in a holistic way, encompassing the biological, psychological, social and organisational domains, with the biological domain referring to the individual's physical issues; the psychological domain corresponds to emotions, reasoning; the social domain refers to family, friends, work colleagues and the organisational domain is associated with aspects of organisational culture, technologies, the size of the organisation, levels of competitiveness in the market (Cavedon, 2014).

Some factors can influence workers' QoL, including stress, pain and accidents at work (Almeida et al., 2014; Golchin et al., 2014). Long working hours and shifts are considered stressors and can interfere with the quality and quantity of work (Wagstaff, Segstad, 2011); in addition to other factors such as: the precariousness of work, considered by the author Padilha (2009) and understood as flexibility in hiring workers; informalisation of work; outsourcing and fourth outsourcing; strategic turnover, among others mentioned above, can therefore alter and affect workers' QoL.

There are currently instruments that assess some aspects of QoL, which were used in this study. However, no studies have yet been found in the literature evaluating control demand, QoL and sleep in industrial workers at the same time.

The WHOQOL-bref has been used as an important tool for assessing QoL in various populations around the world, including workers from different occupations. Among the different populations assessed, some authors have investigated the relationship between depression and its relationship with the WHOQOL-bref index in healthcare workers in Taiwan and Brazil (Lu et al., 2011; Rios et al., 2010).

Authors have assessed the perception of QoL in dentists and teachers respectively (Penteado, Pereira, 2007). However, in Brazil, only one study was found that characterised QoL in

Brazilian workers in the industrial context, but this research did not relate sleep and control demand, but rather the work ability index (Costa et al., 2012).

However, the evaluation associated with these three indicators can provide a greater understanding of work factors and broader aspects of life related to perceived losses. Also, breaking down this analysis by age group can help identify the most critical aspects and the most vulnerable groups, which in turn can help determine more effective control measures.

The health of workers involved in various factors including the manufacturing sector in India deserves attention for safety and productivity, there are several existing risks, including physical risks, as well as psychosocial risks (Suri, Das, 2016).

Quality of life can be impacted in the physical domain due to heatwave stress and can trigger work accidents; heat stress can induce other construction accidents due to physical fatigue, impaired mental capacity and poor use of mental impaired mental capacity and poor use of personal protective equipment (PPE) (Rameezdeen, Elmualim , 2017).

In addition to the hazards encountered on the construction site, construction workers are also subjected to physical and chemical risks (e.g. dust, powders, fibres, noise), among others, throughout the process, and these risks can affect the worker and still interfere with Quality of Life (Yi, Chan, 2017).

Work-related injuries to the upper limbs account for the majority of occupational illnesses, sleep apnoea syndrome, a consequent decrease in quality of life and with mood disorders, obesity, decreased productivity, limited ability and risks of accidents at work (Golchin et al., 2014, Jurado-Gomez et al., 2014).

Some factors can interfere with quality of life, mainly reflecting on the worker's physical health, such as back pain, fatigue, muscle pain, health and tobacco use are associated with outsourced contracts, however there is little research on the relationship between outsourced contracts and formal work, in the case of this thesis the contract regulated by the Consolidation of Labour Laws (CLT) (Alali et al., 2016).

Stress has been associated with anxiety and depression, and anxiety and depression are associated with poor quality of life (Teles et al., 2014)

There are currently instruments that can assess some aspects of quality of life, which were used in this study. However, no studies have yet been found in the literature evaluating control demand, quality of life and sleep in industrial workers at the same time.

CHAPTER 3

Methodological considerations

This is an exploratory, cross-sectional, descriptive study with a quantitative approach among outsourced construction workers. The main hypothesis of this study is that injured construction workers have worse QoL scores, lower demand for control and less sleep than healthy workers.

The study was carried out in a petrochemical industry built in the 1950s, located in the town of Cubatão/SP. This unit has been undergoing alterations and adjustments since 2007, due to existing environmental legislation, with the aim of reducing the emission of gases contained in fuels, both petrol and diesel.

For this modernisation to take place, companies are hired by the petrochemical industry in the form of contracts and subcontracts with firms in the construction industry, where workers in a wide variety of jobs, such as welders, bricklayers and scaffolding erectors, are carrying out their activities. The form of contract is by employment under the Consolidation of Labour Laws (CLT) and by service providers who make up the group of aggregates (Brasil, 1943).

Working hours are eight hours, Monday to Saturday, with one day off per week. Daytime work starts at 7.30am and ends at 5.30pm with one hour's rest; night-time work starts at 7pm and ends at 7am the following day, with one hour's rest.

Participants were those who had suffered accidents at work, with or without time off work (Law 8213/1991). And for healthy workers, i.e. those not affected by accidents at work, the three questionnaires were distributed randomly at the Occupational Health Outpatient Clinic (Brasil, 1991). Workers who had suffered commuting accidents and were on holiday, on medical leave or on pregnancy leave were excluded. All outsourced construction workers who had suffered typical accidents at work (n = 29) and the same number of healthy outsourced workers (n = 29) took part, totalling 58 outsourced workers, between 1st July 2013 and 1st July 2013.

2014, belonging to both day and night shifts. However, in this survey, no night workers were affected by OA and healthy workers did not answer the questionnaire. The average number of outsourced workers in this period was 4,118.

The non-probabilistic sampling technique was used, considering that the criteria adopted in the study were workers who had been affected by an accident at work, and the same number of healthy workers, except for those belonging to the exclusion criteria, where their number was informed, if any.

This research was carried out in accordance with the guidelines and regulatory standards set out in Resolution 466/12, belonging to the National Health Council, approved under

CEP/UNIFESP number 319253. All participants signed the Free and Informed Consent Form (Brasil, 2012). Appendix A.

The workers who answered the questionnaires belonged to construction trades such as scaffolders and sanders, except for one employee who worked as a cook in one of the three restaurants located within the study site.

In order to develop this thesis, we analysed 3 complex work instruments that allowed us to correlate many variables of quality of life, sleep and demand control and social support, i.e. psychosocial aspects in the work environment, as described below:

a) Demands Control and Social Support at Work

The DCSQ model, a shortened version of the Job Strain Model questionnaire (Appendix B), contains 17 multiple-choice questions, subdivided into three scales: I - control at work and decision-making: six questions about work - questions about control at work and questions about decision-making); II - demands at work: five questions about demands at work (these are about time and speed to do the job) and III - social support in the work environment: six questions about social support that the worker receives in their work environment (Alves et al, 2015; Magnano et al., 2010b).

The questionnaire was administered by the research nurse after the worker had been seen in the unit's emergency department, when possible, or when the worker was able to answer the 17 questions with response options for the "psychological demand" and "control" dimensions, which were presented on a *Likert-type* scale (1-4), ranging from "often" to "never/almost never". Each answer was given a score from 1 to 4, considering items with a reverse score on both scales (Alves et al., 2015; Magnano et al., 2010b).

The scores were obtained in two ways: one was quantitative, where they were obtained by adding up the items in each dimension and ranged from 5-20 (demand) and 6-24 (control and social support). High demand, high control and high social support were categorised with values higher than the median for the 58 respondents (11, 11 and 22) and for the 29 injured and healthy respondents (12.10, 11, 12, 24 and 21 respectively); the other, according to the midpoint of the scales, i.e. the scores were obtained by adding up the items in each dimension and ranged from 5-20 (demand) and 6-24 (control and social support). High demand, high control and high social support were categorised into individuals with scores higher than the midpoint of the scale 12.5, 15 and 12.5; low demand high control - make up low demand, low demand low control - passive work; high demand and high control - active work; high demand and low control - high demand, respectively, of construction workers (Alves et al., 2015; Magnano et al., 2010a).

The combination of responses with high control over the work process generates high wear and tear (job strain), causing harmful effects on workers' health. Also harmful to workers' health is the situation in which low demands and low control are combined (passive labour), which can lead to a loss of skills and disinterest. On the other hand, when high demands and low controls coexist, individuals experience the active work process, a situation that is less harmful to workers, since they have the autonomy to choose how to plan their work activities, according to their rhythm. The ideal low-wear situation combines low demands and high control of the work process (Alves et al., 2004). This situation can still result in better sleep quality and less fatigue, but in a situation of low to high fatigue, there is a worsening of sleep quality and an increase in fatigue (Ulhôa, Moreno, 2009).

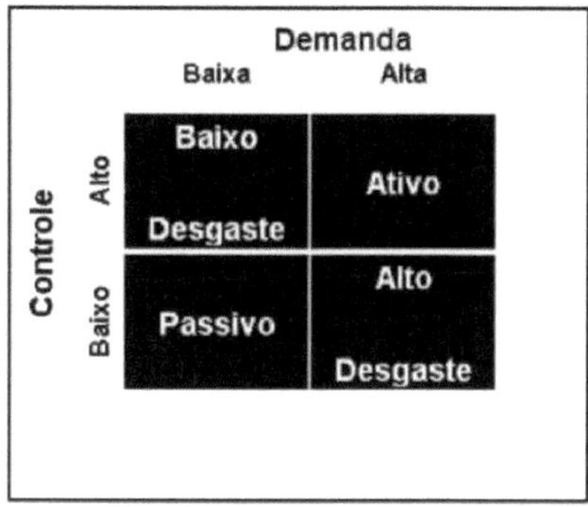

Source: Alves et al. (2004).

Figure 1 - Demand Control Model

b) Quality of Life Questionnaire

In order to assess the perception of QoL among construction workers, the second instrument used was the questionnaire developed by the World Health Organisation Quality of Life Group, the WHOQOL-bref (Annex 2). This instrument has been tested and validated in various cultures, under the coordination of the World Health Organisation Quality of Life Group (WHOQOL GROUP) of the World Health Organisation (WHO). It is a self-administered instrument that considers the last 15 days lived by the respondents and consists of 26 questions, two of which are general. One refers to LIFE and the other to HEALTH and is not included in the equations used to analyse the results. The remaining twenty-four questions relate to the four domains and their respective facets that make up the original instrument.

The physical domain focuses on the following facets: pain and discomfort, energy and fatigue, sleep and rest, activities of daily living, dependence on medication or treatment, ability to work; the psychological domain includes the facets: positive feelings, thinking, learning, memory and concentration, self-esteem, body image and appearance, negative feelings, spirituality, religiosity and personal beliefs; the social relations domain includes the facets: social support, sexual activity; and the environmental domain includes the facets: positive feelings, thinking, learning, memory and concentration, self-esteem, body image and appearance, negative feelings, spirituality, religiosity and personal beliefs.

following facets: physical safety and security, home environment, financial resources, health and social care, availability and quality, opportunities to acquire new information and skills, participation in, and opportunities for recreation/leisure, physical environment with pollution, noise, traffic, climate, transport.

To calculate the WHOQL- bref instrument, the answers are made up of five optional items on likert-type scales ranging from one to five points. The results of the domains have values between zero and one hundred, the worst being those closest to zero and the best being those closest to 100 (one hundred).

The intensity scale ranges from not at all to extremely; the capacity scale from not at all to completely; the evaluation scale from very satisfied to very dissatisfied and very bad to very good and the frequency scale ranges from never to always. All the facets have answers from 1 to 5, and in questions 3, 4 and 26, the scores are inverted according to 1=5; 2=4, 3=3, 4=2, 5=1. The two facets Q1 and Q2 assess general QoL and are calculated together to generate a single score, independent of the domain scores.

c) Munich Chronotype Questionnaire

The third instrument is the Munich Chronotype Questionnaire (MCTQ), which contains 17 questions (Appendix 3) to assess each individual's sleep profile, based on their sleep phase (Roenneberg et al., 2004). The MCTQ asks about sleep habits, separating days off from days at work (MSF) (Roenneberg et al., 2004). A sleep deficit is expected to be compensated for on free days, so the MSF is corrected for working days, resulting in the MSFsc of local time. This tool classifies the chronotype according to the population to which it belongs.

According to Allebrandt and Roenneberg (2008), the MCTQ questionnaire provides a quantitative measure of average sleep time. The MSFsc does not have scores, but its result is obtained by means of a continuous distribution approximating a normal curve, with the chronotypes with extreme values being the afternoon and morning chronotypes, and minimum limits of 30 per cent of the values of each population assessed are used for this population.

Statistical analysis

Correlations between quantitative variables were carried out using Spearman's correlation coefficient (Pagano, Gauvreau, 2004). This coefficient is non-parametric and ranges from -1 to 1, where values closer to -1 indicate a negative or inverse relationship between the variables; values close to 1, a positive relationship and values close to 0 indicate no correlation.

Comparisons between the groups with regard to quantitative variables were made using the unpaired Student's t-test for variables with a normal distribution in each of the groups; and using the Mann-Whitney non-parametric test (Pagano, Gauvreau, 2004) for variables where this assumption was not met.

Internal consistency was analysed using Chronbach's alpha coefficient (1951), which ranges from 0 to 1 and where values greater than 0.7 indicate reliability between the measures (Martins, 2006).

For all the analyses, a significance level of 5% and the Statistical Analysis System (SAS) version 9.2 software were used.

CHAPTER 4

Results and Discussion

The following are the results obtained among construction workers, whose average age among the 58 workers was 35.6. ± 10.6.

Table 1 shows that the majority of the sample (98.2%) belonged to the male sex, with non-smoking workers in both groups (82.7%) (Table 1).

When compared to smoking, with the same number of individuals, it was found in both groups (82.7 per cent), respectively.

Table 1. Distribution of samples by gender, age group and tobacco use. Cubatão - SP, 2015

Variable		Total	Healthy	Accident victims
Age (years)		35,66±10.69	33,10±10,10(n=29)	38,21±10,81(n=29)
Sex	Female	1,72% (n=1)	0%(n=0)	3,45%(n=1)
	Male	98,28% (n=57)	100%(n=29)	96,55%(n=28)
Smoking	Yes	17,24%(n=48)	17,24%(n=5)	17,24%(n=5)
	No	82,76%(n=10)	82,76%(n=24)	82,76%(n=24)

Today's working life is characterised by incessant rhythms, the intensification of production regimes and urgent changes. In addition to these structural changes, the current economic crisis is putting increasing pressure on employers and workers to maintain adequate levels of competitiveness. Many of these changes offer opportunities for development, but at the same time can increase psychosocial risks and negative effects on QoL, with repercussions on health and safety.

In this study, males predominated, a characteristic of the profession of construction workers. Several studies have also shown a predominance of males (Ferraz, Aquino, 2014; Abas et al., 2013; Lykouras et al., 2014; Garg et al., 2012; Mejia et al., 2015).

The average age of construction workers who work during the day among the injured was 38.2 years (Serkalem et al., 2014). Another study also found average age values among workers in a construction industry similar to the present study, however, among the injured and those with some kind of occupational disease, which was similar to the present study, totalling an average age of 42.3 years (Brito, 2007; Lykouras et al., 2014;).

Table 2 shows the workers' jobs in terms of the healthy and injured groups, with the majority being fitters (24.13 per cent of the healthy and 17.34 per cent of the injured); 10.34 per cent being plumbers in both groups; 10.34 per cent being sanders among the healthy and 3.44 per cent among the injured; 6.89 per cent being mechanics among the healthy and 6.89 per cent being carpenters and belonging to both groups of workers.

Table 2. Distribution of the sample in terms of the injured and healthy groups. Cubatão - SP, 2015

Functions	Healthy n		Accident victims	
		%	n	%
Administrative	2	6,89%	1	3,44%
Plumber	3	10,34%	3	10,34%
Welder	2	6,89%	0	0
Assembler	7	24,13%	5	17,26%
Grinder	3	10,34%	1	3,44%
Mechanic	2	6,89%	0	0
Carpenter	2	6,89%	2	6,89%
Not informed In the Instrument	6	20,70%	4	13,80%
Cook	0	0	2	6,89%
Others	2	6,89%	11	37,94%

In this study, there was a predominance of workers who did not smoke, results similar to those found in the studies by Galdino et al., 2012; Serkalem et al., 2014.

All the outsourced construction workers who took part in this study are employed under the Consolidation of Labour Laws (CLT). The predominant profession among the healthy and injured workers was fitter.

Human labour is an integral part of infrastructure growth and people who work on construction sites are at great risk to their health, as the construction sector is considered one of the risk sectors due to the characteristics to which these workers are exposed, such as working at height, handling heavy and bulky equipment, as well as high temperatures with cotton clothing which, in summer, can also provide a risk of dehydration and lipothymia. Exposure of these workers to conditions such as those mentioned above can lead to physical and psychological stress, a reduction in their attention threshold and a risk of accidents (Tomei et al., 2015, Basnet et al., 2010).

The workers in this study work fixed hours, but during periods when the work schedule is being carried out, they can work overtime and also, if they need to be hired, shift work.

The hours worked by construction workers, eight (8) hours a day with two hours of overtime, are similar to research carried out in the United States and the Netherlands where work up to 60 and 70 hours a week respectively (Wagstaff, Segstad, 2011; Tomei et al., 2015). Long working hours and shift workers contribute to a relative increase in the risk of accidents and other similar events that can occur in various areas, including construction. For example, in a study carried out in an oil company, with variable 8-hour shifts, the accident rate was higher when compared to fixed-shift workers (Almeida et al., 2014; Tomei et al., 2015; Wagstaff, Segstad, 2011; Brito, 2007).

In addition to the daily working hours, it is important to note that working hours are between 7.30am and 5.30pm, with the exception of overtime. When workers work overtime, this can extend to 7.30pm. Working in the early hours of the morning can affect alertness and performance. The lack of synchronisation with the temperature curve and cortisol levels can increase the risk of accidents. All accidents at work occurred during the daytime, from seven to ten o'clock, corroborating the literature which says that accidents are likely to occur from nine to eleven o'clock, with a decreased likelihood of occurring at lunchtime. This data was taken from a survey of workers building tunnels in Iran. Major accidents have occurred as a result of tiredness and the time of day when activities were carried out, such as the Three Mile Island accidents, the Exxon Valdez oil spill, where everything happened between midnight and 6am. These accidents, along with a large number of transport accidents on roads and in construction, have been linked to human fatigue (Fischer et al., 2000; Fossum et al., 2013, Haghighi, Yazdi, 2015, Tomei et al., 2015; Amiri , Ardeshir , Zarandi, 2015).

The workers in this study compensated for their sleep deficit with longer periods of sleep. This situation was also observed in a study in which masons and bricklayers showed a greater need for sleep recovery than the general working population, because they are subjected to a high pace of work. Therefore, the need for sleep recovery after work can be a sign of mental and physical fatigue and is considered a predictor of adverse health effects (Haghighi, Yazdi, 2015, Tomei et al., 2015).

It has been observed that shift workers have at least three nocturnal awakenings, while workers with fixed working hours find it more difficult to wake up (Tomei et al., 2015).

Even though the injured workers in this research did not work shifts, it is essential to address in this thesis relevant data from a study by Tomei et al., 2015, in which police workers who work shifts have a higher incident rate of 72% compared to the day shift and 66% compared to the afternoon shift. The incidence remains consistently high throughout the working week because of poor quality and quantity of sleep, as well as increased physical and mental fatigue.

Overtime, job dissatisfaction, anxiety and stress can have a negative influence on workers' attitudes and thus contribute to accidents at work (Tomei et al., 2015), Regarding the perception of QoL, 51.72% of workers rated their QoL as good, 32% as very good, 13.7% as neither good nor bad and 1% as bad (Table 3).Regarding the second question, how satisfied are you with your QoL, 41.3% said they were satisfied, 39.6% were very satisfied, 8.6% were neither satisfied nor dissatisfied, 6.9% were dissatisfied and 3.4% were very satisfied. It can be seen that 39.6% of those interviewed were aged 30 or under, 27.5% between 31 and 40, 20.6% between 41 and 50 and 12.0% between 51 and 60.

Table 3. Distribution of the sample regarding questions 1 and 2 of the Whoqol-bref, age group, gender and tobacco use. Cubatão - SP, 2015

Variable	n	%

Whoqol 1		
Bad	1	1,72
Neither bad nor good	8	13,79
Good	30	51,72
Very good	19	32,76
Whoqol 2		
Very dissatisfied	2	3,45
Unsatisfactory	4	6,90
Not satisfied Not satisfied	5	8,62
Satisfied	24	41,38
Very satisfied	23	39,66
Sex		
Female	1	1,72
Male	57	98,28
Smoking		
No	48	82,76
Yes	10	17,24
Age group		
<= 30	23	39,66
31 a 40	16	27,59
41 a 50	12	20,69
51 a 60	7	12,07

With regard to the QoL of construction workers, the survey showed that the social domain received the best evaluation, followed by the psychological and environmental domains. The physical domain had lower scores, but the majority of workers rated their health as good and were satisfied.

Figure 2 shows the minimum values for the first quartile, median, third quartile and maximum values for the four QoL domains. The physical domain had the worst average, 63.52%; followed by the environmental domain, 62.5%; psychological, 67.2% and the social domain, which had the best average, 81%.

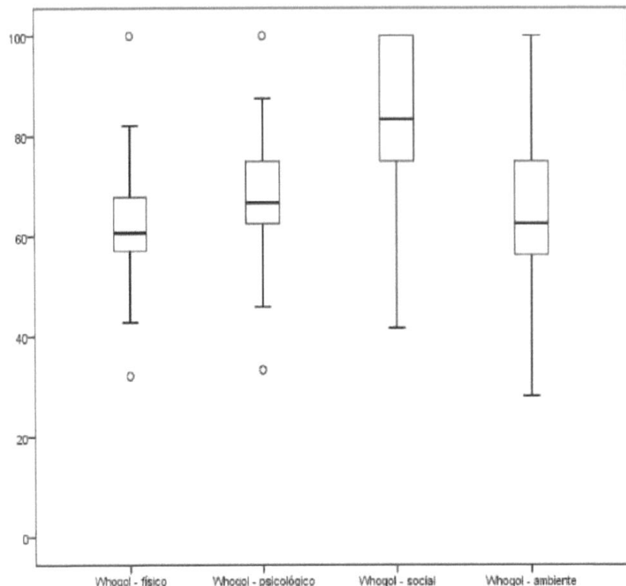

Figure 2. Distribution of Quality of Life domains. Cubatão - SP, 2015

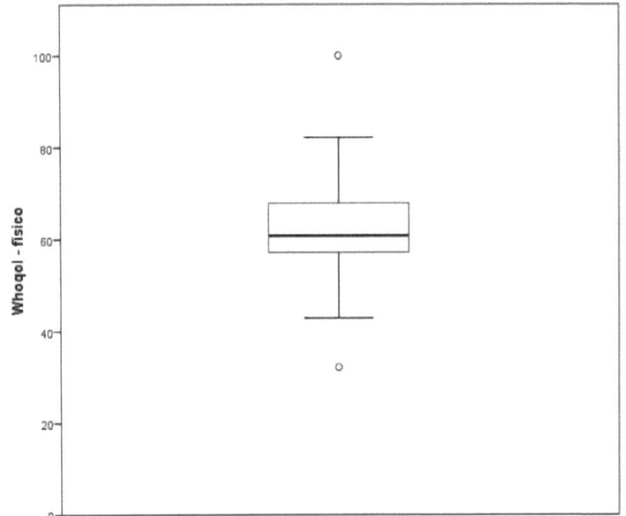

Figure 3 - Distribution of the Physical domain. Cubatão - SP, 2015

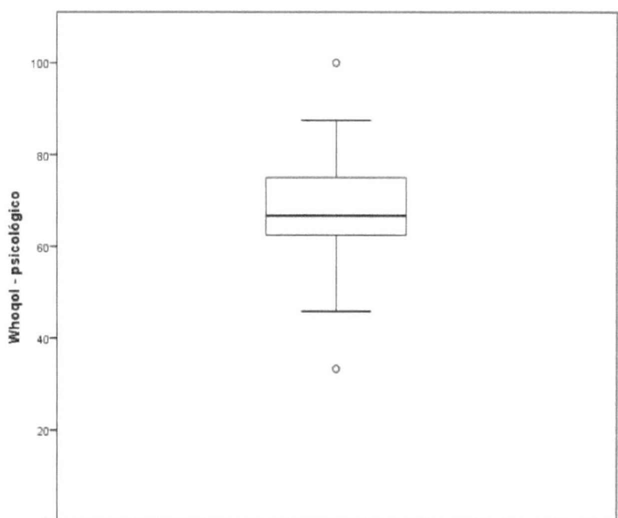

Figure 4 - Distribution of the Psychological domain. Cubatão - SP, 2015

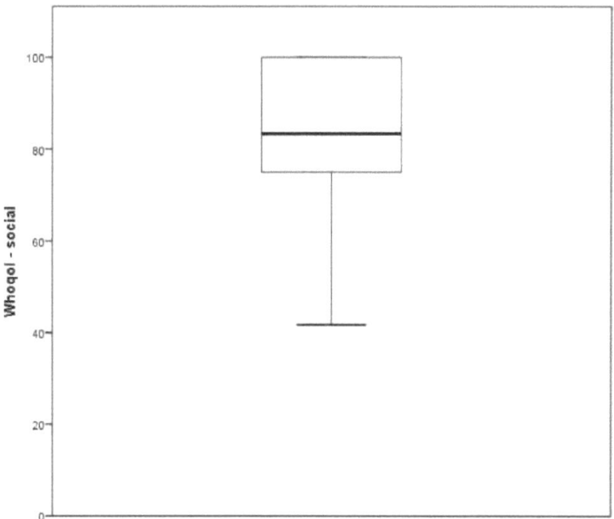

Figure 5 - Distribution of the Social domain. Cubatão - SP, 2015

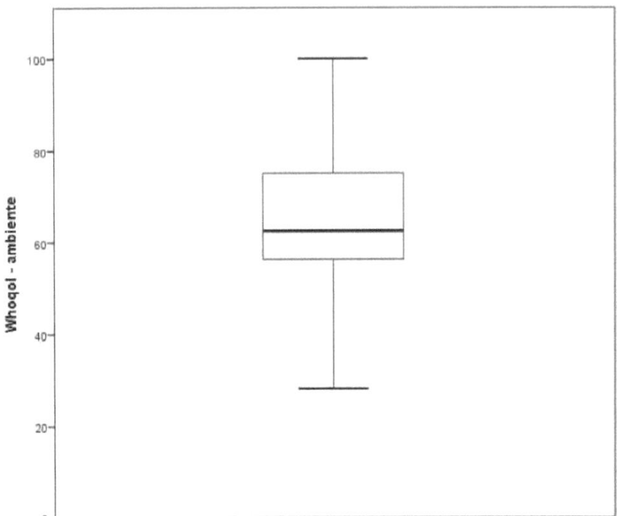

Figure 6. Distribution of the Environment domain. Cubatão - SP, 2015

When analysing the scores for each domain and the self-assessment of QoL, it can be seen that the average value was low in the physical domain. This situation can be attributed to accidents at work in which workers show some kind of physical deterioration as a result of the existing injury.

It can also be said that construction workers suffer from many musculoskeletal problems, such as lumbar sacral algias, due to the enormous wear and tear and physical effort they put in on a daily basis, which is often chronic (Jacobsen et al., 2013).

In addition to the factors that involve the characteristics of the physical work environment, workers can currently also be pressurised to comply with the stages of the work, according to Magnussum et al., 2014. This situation can lead to psychological problems and an unhealthy working environment.

Despite the relevance of the subject of QoL in construction workers, few studies are published in the scientific community, which makes it difficult to compare whether the workers in this study have a worse or better QoL. However, when compared with the study by Costa et al., 2012, among workers in the school materials industry, the results were different. The worst domain in this study was the physical domain in the total sample, unlike the environmental domain in the aforementioned study.

It can be seen that when comparing healthy and injured workers during the day, the averages of the QoL domains were evaluated, with the physical domain having the worst average among the injured workers; but among the healthy workers, the worst average was the environmental domain, with a significant difference. However, it can be said that the social relations domain in both groups showed the best averages.

The average duration of sleep on working days, between Monday and Friday, was 10 hours (the average duration of half the sleep was 5 hours and 33 minutes). When we looked at the average duration of sleep on days off, between Saturday and Sunday, it was 18 hours and 33 minutes and the average duration of half the sleep on days off was 9 hours, therefore higher values. The average duration of general sleep was 12 hours and 18 minutes and the average duration of half of general sleep was 6 hours and 8 minutes. The average social jet lag (difference between the midpoint of sleep on days off compared to days at work) was 13 hours and 16 minutes and the average for how many days of regular hours was 5.6 minutes (Table 4).

The average scores for the physical, psychological and environmental domains were between 62.3, 67.2 and 63.5, with the average obtained for the social domain being the highest at 81.

The average scores found for social demand were 11.4, for control 11.7 and for social support 21.1.

Table 4: Values of sleep variables, quality of life domains and control demand according to sample characteristics. Cubatão - SP, 2015.

Variable	n	Mediuma	Deviation-standard	Minimum	Q1	Mediana	Q3	Maximum
Age	58	35,66	10,69	19,00	26,00	34,00	42,00	58,00
Quantity of cigarettes	10	10,40	5,30	3,00	5,00	11,00	15,00	17,00
Sleep duration - working day	51	10,00	11,50	0,16	3,00	0,73	23,15	23,91
Half sleep - working day	51	5,33	5,75	0,08	0,16	0,36	11,82	11,95
Sleep duration - day off	47	18,13	9,90	0,16	23,00	23,50	23,75	24,00
Half sleep - day off	47	9,00	4,95	0,08	11,33	11,75	11,86	12,00
Sleep duration - general	53	12,18	10,30	0,01	0,65	7,00	23,56	23,91
Half sleep - general	53	6,08	5,15	0,08	0,32	3,53	11,70	11,95
Jet lag	53	13,16	9,48	5,00	0,50	12,00	23,45	23,91
How many days reg.	58	5,62	0,67	5,00	5,00	6,00	6,00	7,00

Whoqol -Q1	58	4,16	0,72	2,00	4,00	4,00	5,00	5,00
Whoqol -Q2	58	4,07	1,04	1,00	4,00	4,00	5,00	5,00
Whoqol - physicist	58	62,38	10,52	32,14	57,14	60,71	67,86	100,00
Whoqol - psychological	58	67,24	10,57	33,33	62,50	66,67	75,00	100,00
Whoqol - social	58	81,03	16,43	41,67	75,00	83,33	100,00	100,00
Whoqol - environment	58	63,52	16,01	28,13	56,25	62,50	75,00	100,00
Demand	58	11,43	3,70	6,00	9,00	11,00	14,00	20,00
Control	58	11,74	3,35	6,00	9,00	11,00	14,00	22,00
Social support	58	21,16	3,46	11,00	20,00	22,00	24,00	24,00

The QoL results indicated an average score of 70.15 for the environment domain for workers in the injured group and an average of 56.90 for workers in the healthy group. There was also a median score of 71.88 for the injured group of workers and a median score of 59.38 for the healthy group. The unpaired Student's t-test showed a significant difference between the two groups in terms of the mean values for this domain ($p<0.05$). (Table 5).

For the demand variable, the results indicated a mean of 12.97 for the group of injured workers and a mean of 9.90 for the group of healthy workers. As well as median values of 12.00 for the injured group and a median of 10.00 for the healthy group, a significant difference was observed between the two groups with regard to the mean values of this variable ($p<0.05$).

For social support, mean values of 21.93 were found for the injured group and a mean of 20.38 for the healthy group. As well as a median of 24 in the injured group and a median of 21 in the healthy group, there was a significant difference between the two groups with regard to the mean values of the demand variable ($p<0.05$).

Table 5. Comparison of injured and healthy workers in terms of perceived quality of life and control demand variables. Cubatão - SP, 2015.

Variables	Healthy	n	Accident victims	n	p-value
Domain	61,70±12.40	29	63,05±8,39	29	0,6283

Physical Domain	65,09±12.47	29	69,40±7,90	29	0,225
Psychological Relationships	77,59±17.97	29	84,88±14,21	29	0,1490**
Social Duration	14,08±10.48	29	10,06±9,91	29	0,2310**
Sleep Domain	56,90±16.27	29	70,15±12,9	29	**0,0011**
Environment					
Demand	9,90±2.88	29	12,97±3,82	29	**0,0011**
Control	11,58±2,32	29	11,9±4,18	29	0,7027**
Social Support	20,38±3.38	29	21,93±3,41	29	**0,0089**

Note: * p-value obtained using the unpaired Student's t-test.

1 p-value obtained using the Mann-Whitney test.

Table 6 shows negative correlations between sleep variables and perceived QoL, showing that the more hours of sleep a worker has, the lower their perceived QoL, when related to the physical domain (r = - 0.41).

It was found that individuals slept more during working days and had a worse perception of QoL in the physical and environmental domains. The amount of sleep and QoL may be related to fatigue and/or sleep disturbances, and could therefore impair performance during working hours. It is also important to note that the physical agents and stressors present in an organisation, added to environmental agents such as the high noise inherent in industrial areas, can impair sleep (Feder et al., 2015, Oliveira et al., 2015).

The highest Jet Leg Social values occurred when sleep time was shorter. The perception of these individuals was also worse (r= -0.29).

It was observed that the longer the duration of sleep on regular working days, the lower the perception of the environmental domain (r= -0.34), thus expressing a weak correlation between the variables.

Table 6. Correlation between sleep variables and Quality of Life. Cubatão - SP, 2015.

Variables	**Sample Total**		
	n	**P**	**r**
Sleep Duration - Day Off X Physical	47	**0,0041**	-0,41*
Social X Physical Jet Lag	53	**0,0349**	-0,29*
Sleep Duration - Regular Working Day X Environment	58	**0,0091**	-0,34*

1 Spearman's correlation test;

In Table 7, the correlation values show that the higher the demand values, the shorter the sleep time, with a statistically significant difference (r= - 0.27) according to Spearman's test.

Table 7. Correlation between sleep duration on working days and Demand Control Domain Scores. Cubatão - SP, 2015.

Variables	Sample Total		
	n	P	r
Sleep Duration X Demand	58	**0,0406**	-0,27*
Sleep Duration X Control	58	0,0687	-0,24*
Sleep Duration X Social Support	58	0,0322	-0,13*

* Spearman's correlation test;

In the total sample of workers, short sleep duration was observed when high work demands coexist, a similar situation observed in research by Magnussum et al., 2014.

Table 8 shows that the higher the perception of the physical domain, the higher the perception of the psychological domain (r=0.27, p=0.417) and (r=0.55, p=<0.0001).

The psychological domain showed a correlation with the social domain (r=0.44 p=0.0006) and the environmental domain (r=0.45, p=0.0004).

The highest correlation observed was between the social domain and the environmental domain (r= 0.57).

A positive correlation was observed between the four QoL domains. There was a moderate correlation between the social domain and the other domains, and between the psychological and environmental domains.

Table 8. Correlation between the physical, psychological, social and environmental domains of workers Cubatão - SP, 2015.

Variables	Sample Total		
	n	P	r
Physical X Psychological	58	**0,0417**	0,27*
Physical X Social	58	**<0,0001**	0,55*
Physical X Environmental	58	0,1005	0.22*
Psychological X Social	58	**0,0006**	0,44*
Psychological X Environmental	58	**0,0004**	0,45*

Social X Environmental	58	**<0,0001**	0,57*

1 Spearman's correlation test;

The correlation between the four QoL domains was positive, showing that there is a moderate correlation between the social domain and the other domains, and between the psychological and environmental domains.

It was observed that the higher the perception of the physical domain, the greater the social support among construction workers (r=0.28, p=0.0345);

It can also be seen that the higher the perception of the psychological domain, the greater the social support among workers (r=0.35, p=<0.0077);

The higher social domain is related to greater social support among workers (r=0.38, p=0.0036);

The lower environmental domain is related to higher demand among workers (r=0.36, p=0.0059), a medium correlation.

The higher environmental domain is related to greater social support among workers (r=0.39, p=0.0023).

The social support variable was found to have positive correlations with the QoL variables in the physical (r=0.28), psychological (r=0.35) and social (r=0.38) domains, showing that this is an important factor in the perception of QoL. Among the demand variable we can see that there was a positive correlation with the environmental domain (r=0.36), the same occurring with social support (r=0.39) (Table 9).

Table 9. Correlation between the physical, psychological, social and environmental domains of workers X Demand Control. Cubatão - SP, 2015.

Variables	Sample Total		
	n	P	r
Physical X Demand	58	0,5312	-0,08*
Physical X Control	58	0,8193	-0,03*
Physical X Social Support	58	0,0345	0,28*
Psychological X Demand	58	0,5507	-0,08*
Psychological X Control	58	0,9965	0,00*
Psychological	58	<0,0077	0,35*

X Social support			
Social X Demand	58	0,3796	0,12*
Social X Control	58	0,2004	0,17*
Social X Social Support	58	0,0036	0,38*
Environment X Demand	58	0,0059	0,36*
Environment X Control	58	0,1789	0,17*
Environment X Social Support	58	0,0023	0,39*

* p-value obtained using the unpaired Student's t-test.Spearman;

There was a moderate correlation between the environment and work demands, which allows us to say that work demands among construction workers are inversely related to the environment, a similar situation observed among metalworkers in Malaysia; there was no significant correlation in control when correlated with social support; however, control is related to social relationships in a study by Rusli, Edimansyah, Naing L, 2008.

Table 10 shows that the correlations between the demand-control and social support variables are significant. The values of (r=0.41, p=0.0014), average correlation, performed by Spearman's correlation test. The other correlations showed no statistically significant difference.

The correlation between the demand for control and social support variables was positive (r=0.41).

Social support is correlated with the Physical, Psychological and Social domains, so an increase in social support predicts higher perceptions of the four dimensions of QoL, a similar situation found in the study carried out by Rusli, Edimansyah, Naing L, 2008.

Among this group of construction workers surveyed, demand is correlated with social support, i.e. the lower the demand, the greater the social support among workers in the workplace, making for a favourable condition, a similar situation among Swedish workers; however, a lack of social support can lead to symptoms of insecurity and fear of losing one's job (Magnussum et al., 2014; Tomei et al., 2015).

In this study, there was no correlation between control and QoL domains. In a study by Magnussum et al., 2014, it was observed that work control is directly related to the physical health, psychological health and social relationships domains of the WHOQOL-BREF.

It was observed that the greater the demand, the greater the social support among employees, with values higher than the median 11.

Table 10. Correlation between Demand Control variables. Cubatão - SP, 2015.

Variables	Sample Total		
	n	P	r
Demand X Control	58	0,0881	0,23*
Demand X Social support	58	**0,0014**	0,41*
Control X Social support	58	0,7049	0,05*

* Spearman's correlation test;

Among the injured workers, sleep duration on working days, when correlated with days off, showed no correlation. For the healthy group, there was a correlation showing that the longer the duration of sleep on working days, the longer the sleep time on days off (r= 0.53, p=0.0052). (Table 11).

Sleep duration on working days, when correlated with general sleep, allows us to say that the longer the sleep time on working days, the longer the average daily sleep duration in both groups.

Workers in the injured and healthy groups slept less (r=0.53, p=0.0052).

It can also be seen that when correlated, the duration of sleep on days off is longer and this is observed in both groups (r=0.59, p=0.0059) and (r=0.76, p=< 0.0001), a medium and strong correlation respectively.

With regard to sleep duration on days off (Saturday and Sunday, or Sunday only), compared to social jet lag, both injured and healthy workers slept more to compensate for the sleep debt that was acquired during the week ($p<0.05$).

Table 11. Correlation between sleep variables in the injured and healthy worker groups. Cubatão - SP, 2015

Variables	Accident victims		Healthy	
Sleep Duration	P	r	P	r
- Working Day X	0,5805	0,14*	**0,0052**	0,53*

Day Off Sleep Duration - Labour Day X AVSD	**0,0422**	0,42*	**< 0,0001**	0,92*
Sleep Duration - Working Day X Social Jet Lag	**0,0146**	0,49*	**< 0,0001**	0,86*
Sleep Duration - Working Day X Regular Hours	0,1168	0,33*	0,3954	0,17*
Sleep Duration - Day Off X AVSD	**0,0059**	0,59*	**< 0,0001**	0,76*
Sleep Duration - Day Off X Social Jet Lag	**0,0072**	0,58*	**< 0,0001**	0,85*
Sleep Duration - General X Social Jet Lag	**< 0,0001**	0,91*	**< 0,0001**	0,95*

*Spearman's correlation test;

Table 12 shows that there is a correlation between the domains for analysing QoL, whose data showed statistically significant differences using Spearman's correlation test. With values for the physical domain and social relationships in both groups (r=0.58, p=0.001), medium correlation (r=0.45, p=0.0135) for the psychological and social domain among the healthy; (r=0.47, p=0.0089), medium correlation and social for the environmental in both groups; (r=0..73, p=< 0.0001), strong correlation and (r=0.37, p=0.0484), medium correlation.

Table 12. Correlation between the Quality of Life domains of the 2 groups of workers. Cubatão - SP, 2015.

Variables	Accident victims		Healthy	
	P	**r**	**P**	**r**
Physical X Psychological	0,1012	0,31*	0,2755	0,21
Physical X Social Relations	**0,001**	0,58*	**0,0135**	0,45*
Psychological X Social	0,1205	0,29*	**0,0089**	0,47*

Social X Environmental	**< 0,0001**	0,73*	**0,0484**	0,37*

1 p-value obtained using Spearman's unpaired Student's t-test

Figure 7 shows the minimum, first quartile, median, third quartile and maximum values for demand - 6, 9, 11, 14 and 20, control - 6, 9, 11, 14 and 22 and social support - 11, 20, 22, 24 and 24.

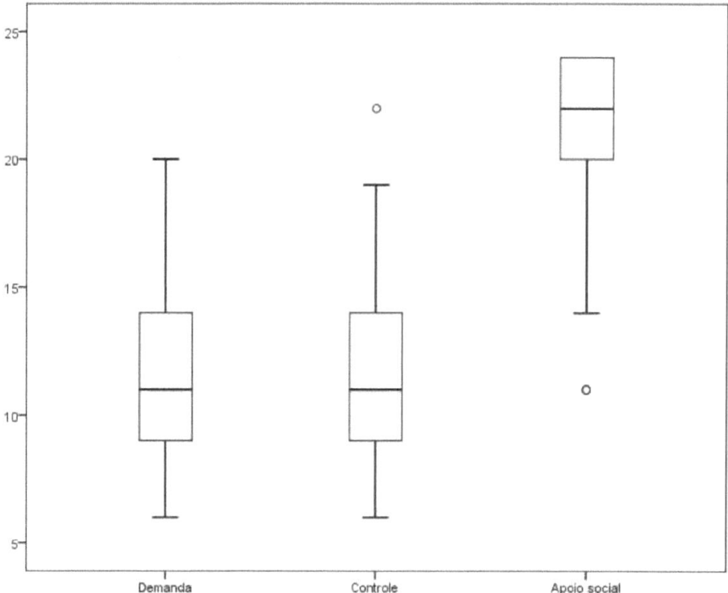

Figure 7- Demand, Control and Social Support values. Cubatão - SP, 2015.

Each category may have professionals with specific stress factors. Workers are always subjected to high levels of stress, with a high incidence of accidents, higher than in other areas. Work in the construction industry is constantly changing and construction workers have to adapt to different environmental and climatic conditions, with notable physical and psychological stress. Accidents are often the result of inattention and carelessness in the preparation of safety measures, due to incessant rhythms, heavy workloads, inadequate training and information. All of these factors are considered to be predictive of stress, which is why it is essential to know the work environment that the worker is exposed to (Tomei et al., 2015).

Construction workers were categorised as having high or low demand, control and social support (values above the midpoint described in the methods above). There was a similarity between healthy and injured workers in terms of demand, where the majority had low demand (82.75%), (51.72%), respectively. The same situation was observed with regard to control (93.10%) among the healthy workers and (79.31%) among the injured workers. Social support was high in both groups (89.65%) and with the same value.

Table 13. Distribution of workers according to classification as high/low demand, control and social support. Cubatão - SP, 2015.

Variables	Category	Healthy	%	Accident victims	%
Demand	Low	24	82,75%	15	51,72%
	High	5	17,25%	14	48,28%
Control	Low	27	93,10%	23	79,31%
	High	2	6,90%	6	20,69%
Social Support	Low	3	10,35%	3	10,35%
	High	26	89,65%	26	89,65%

In addition to the distribution found in table 13, the work of construction workers was categorised according to quadrants in the demand-control model. Only 12% of the healthy workers showed active work and 34.48% of the injured workers; the vast majority of the healthy workers had passive work (87.93%) and just over half (65.71%) of the injured workers.

Table 14. Distribution of workers according to demand-control model categories. Cubatão - SP, 2015.

Variables		Hybrids	%	Accident victims	%
Low demand	↓D C↑	26	44.82%	21	36.20%
Passive Labour	↓D C↓	51	87.93%	38	65.71%
Active Labour	↑D C↑	7	12,00%	20	34.48%
High demand	↑D C↓	32	55,17%	37	63,79%

Psychological demands C= Control

In the correlation between demand control and social support with (r=0.38, p= 0.0442), expressing a moderate correlation, for the other comparisons in the groups analysed, there was no statistically significant difference, as shown in table 15.

Table 15. Correlation between the Demand Control variables between the injured and healthy groups. Cubatão - SP, 2015.

Variables	Accident victims		Healthy	
	P	r	P	r
Demand vs. Control	0,0879	0,32*	0,2032	0,24*
Demand X Social	0,1253	0,29*	**0,0442**	0,38*

Support				
Control X Support Social	0,9842	0,00*	0,8166	0,05*

1 p-value obtained using Spearman's unpaired Student's t-test;

Among the construction workers studied in this research, the results obtained by categorisation showed that the coexistence of low demand and low control were present among injured and healthy construction workers and it is known that the interaction of the two factors - called passive work, intermediate health risk - are seen as inducing a decline in the individual's general activities (Tomei et al., 2015, Magnussum et al., 2014, Prakash et al., 2011).

Therefore, the worker feels apathetic, either due to the lack of new challenges or the absence of decision-making; low control can be translated as a lack of autonomy in the process and can be a psychosocial risk factor and, consequently, for the appearance of depressive symptoms; the low demand present in the study carried out by Tomei et al., 2015 was similar (Tomei et al., 2015, Magnussum et al., 2014, Prakash et al., 2011).

However, in this study, there was a high level of social support among the workers, but its absence can also lead to the appearance of depressive symptoms. In addition to low control, another risk factor for psychosocial illness can be added: low participation in decision-making and lack of support from superiors, which can be evaluated as such and can increase anxiety, stress, mental fatigue and the likelihood of accidents. However, when workers are part of decisions, they feel important and part of the process (Tomei et al., 2015, Magnussum et al., 2014, Prakash et al., 2011).

The level of stress increases if there is no support from colleagues or superiors. In this sense, social isolation and lack of co-operation can increase the risk of work-related stress. On the other hand, carrying out work tasks with a high degree of control in a work environment with social relationships that can guarantee adequate support, contributes to the worker's well-being (Tomei et al., 2015).

Of the demand-control model, the one that is most damaging to workers' health is the high level of demand found in this study, where workers are constantly being asked to perform, but with little participation in the work process (Magnano et al., 2010b).

Construction workers need greater psychophysical recovery after work and, if we analyse, there is an appreciable degree of incidence of depressive syndromes among contractors, whose special work, with adverse conditions, can certainly lead to excessive stress and significant psychological commitment, which are associated with the excessive insecurity that these people are often forced to confront (Tomei et al., 2015).

In addition to the characteristics mentioned above, workers also have characteristics inherent to the process of carrying out a construction project, such as the time it takes to complete the work they have been asked to do, which can also be a trigger for physical and emotional illnesses (Tomei et al., 2015).

Occupational accidents have an important impact on the integrity of the human person and can also bring high costs to a country's social security system and cause increased absenteeism and low productivity, permanent disabilities and deaths (Alizadeh et al., 2015).

CHAPTER 5

Final considerations

The study found a profile for construction workers: male, non-smokers, predominantly fitters and with an average age of 35.6 in the total sample, among injured workers the average age was 38.1 and among healthy workers the average age was 33.1.

The daily hours worked exceeded eight hours, so the work extended into the night shift until around 7.30pm, exhausting the workers.

The research showed that the results of the workers' QoL were best evaluated in the social domain, followed by the psychological and environmental domains. The evaluation of the physical domain showed low scores, due to the injuries caused by accidents at work, although the overall QoL of these workers was considered good.

The environmental domain also obtained a low score and this value can be attributed to basically two situations: the work environment and the place where the workers, who generally come from other parts of Brazil, live, often even without adequate infrastructure.

When the groups were compared, the healthy showed the worst score and the injured the worst domain, which was physical.

Workers have long and exhausting working hours, so they probably sleep more at weekends in an attempt to compensate for the tiredness they generate during the week.

With regard to the psychosocial environment, this study identified greater social support among outsourced construction workers. As a result, there was less demand, even with the characteristic of the employment relationship, which is outsourcing. This is therefore a positive situation, since workers can count on each other, supporting each other and providing a more health-friendly working environment.

The predominant characteristic found in this research was low demand and low control, making for a harmful situation, but high demand and low control was also observed, which is more harmful to the physical and mental health of construction workers.

Therefore, this study indicated the possibility of accidents at work due to the presence of psychosocial and physical factors in the working environment of this population.

Based on my experience as a labour nurse and the development of this research project, I would like to mention some fundamental characteristics of the psychosocial characteristics of work.

It is clear from the references mentioned in this thesis that for workers to be satisfied and committed to their work, they need to be part of it. Being part of it means that workers are inserted into the work context through control over the activities they carry out. Autonomy can provide a much more creative and safe environment for workers and their teams.

Rethinking leadership styles and training managers can be an important tool for improving the psychosocial characteristics of work, thus providing physical and mental health for workers.

We recommend rethinking how daily tasks are delegated to workers, which could be a good strategy for them to be able to set up a more active, more controlled, more democratic workplace, with a consequent interest in training and accident prevention. As a result, the working environment will become much more productive and interesting for supervisors, foremen and site workers in general.

We also believe that with a better working environment for the worker, accidents may even decrease, as the worker will feel part of the process and valued.

References

1. Abas ABL, Mohd-Said DARB, Aziz MMAB, et al. Fatal occupational injuries among non-governmental employees in Malaysia. Am J Ind Med [Internet]. 2013 [cited 2014 Jan 1]; 56(1):65-76. Available from: http://www.ncbi.nlm.nih.gov/pmc/articles/ PMC3505558/
2. Alali H, Magdad AW, Tanja VH, Lutgart B. Work accident victims: a comparison between non-standard and Standard workers in Belgium. International Journal of Occupational and Environmental Health [Internet]. 2016 [cited 2017 April 16]; 22(2):99-106. Available from: https://www.ncbi.nlm.nih.gov/pmc/articles/PMC4984969/
3. Almonte JC, Mena C,, Ortiz S, Osorio JP. Psychiatry and occupational diseases work in Chile: historical and critical review of a complex relationship. Rev. méd. Chile [Internet]. 2016 Dec [cited 2017 14 April]; 144 (12): 15911597. Available from: http://www.scielo.cl/scielo.php?script=sci_arttext&pid=S0034-98872016001200011&lng=pt.Http://dx.doi.org/10.4067/S0034-98872016001200011.

4. Allebrandt KV, Roenneberg T. The search for circadian clock components in humans: new perspectives for association studies. Braz J Med Biol Res [Internet]. 2008 Aug [cited 2015 June 10]; 41(8):716-721. Available from: http://www.scielo.br/ scielo.php?script=sci_arttext&pid=S0100-879X2008000800013&lng=en.
5. Almeida IM, Vilela RAG, Silva AJN, et al. Modelo de Análise e Prevenção de Acidentes-MAPA: ferramenta para a vigilância em Saúde do Trabalhador. Cien Saude Colet [Internet]. 2014 [cited 2015 June 10]; 19(12):4679-88. Available from:

http://www.scielosp.org/pdf/csc/v19n12/1413-8123-csc-19-12-04679.pdf.

6. Almeida JR, Elias ET, Magalhaes MA, et al. Effect of age on the quality of life and health of waste pickers from an association in Governador Valadares, Minas Gerais, Brazil. Cien Saude Coletiva [Internet]. 2009 [cited 2015 Jun 9]; 14(6):2169-80.Available from: http://www.scielosp.org/ pdf/csc/v14n6/24.pdf.

7. Alves MGM, Braga VM, Faerstein, E, et al. Demand-control model of work stress: considerations on different ways of operationalising the exposure variable. Cad. Saúde Pública [internet]. 2015, [cited 2015 June 9]; 31(1):208-212. Available from: http://www.scielosp.org/scielo.php?script=sci_arttext&pid= S0102-311X2015000100208&lng=en&nrm=iso.
8. Alves MGM, Chor D, Faerstein E, et al. Short version of the "job stress scale": adaptation to Portuguese. Rev. Saúde Pública [Internet]. 2004 Apr [cited 2015 June 10]; 38(2):164-71. Available from: http://www.scielosp.org/scielo.php? script=sci_arttext&pid=S0034-89102004000200003&lng=en.
9. Amiri M, Ardeshir A, Zarandi FHF. Risk-based Analysis of Construction Accidents in Iran During2007-2011- Meta Analyze Study Iranian. J Publ Health, [Internet]. 2014 [cited 2015 Sep 4]; 43(4): 507-522. Available from: http://www.ncbi.nlm.nih.gov/pmc/articles/PMC4433733/
10. Anacleto TS, Louzada FM, Pereira EF. Sleep-wake cycle and attention-deficit/hyperactivity disorder. Rev paul paediat [Internet]. 2011 [cited 2017 April 20]; 29(3):437-42. Available from: http://www.scielo.br/pdf/rpp/v29n3/a20v29n3.pdf
11. Araújo DF, Almondes KM. Assessment of sleepiness in university students of different shifts. Psico [Internet]. 2012 [cited 2017 Apri 20]; 17(2):295-302. Available from: http://www.scielo.br/pdf/pusf/v17n2/v17n2a13.pdf
12. Azevedo R C, Ensslin L, Lacerda, RTO, et al. Performance evaluation of the budgeting process: a case study in a construction site. Ambient. constr [Internet]. 2011 [cited 2015 June 9]; 11(1):85-104. Available from: http://www.scielo.br/scielo.php?script=sci_arttext&pid=S1678-86212011000100007& lng=pt&nrm=iso.
13. Basnet P, Gurung S, Pal R, et al. Occupational stress among tunnel workers in Sikkim. Ind Psychlatry J [Internet] 2010 [cited 2015 Sept 4]; 19(1): 13-9. Available from:

http://www.industrialpsychiatry.org/article.asp?issn=0972-6748;year=2010;volume=19;issue=1 ;spage=13;epage=19;aulast=Basnet

14. Bhattacherjee A, Kunar BM. Miners' return to work following injuries in coal mines Med Pr. [Internet] 2016 [cited 2017 April 2017]; 22;67(6):729-742. Available from: https://www.ncbi.nlm.nih.gov/pubmed/28005082
15. Bordoni PHC, Bordoni LS, Silva J deM, Drumond E de F. Use of the capture-recapture method to improve notification of fatal occupational accident records in the city of Belo Horizonte, Minas Gerais, Brazil, 2011. Epidemiol. Serv. Saúde [Internet]. 2016 Mar [cited 2017 16 April]; 25 (1): 85-94. Avaialable from in: http://www.scielo.br/scielo.php?script=sci_arttext&pid=S2237-96222016000100085&lng=pt.Http://dx.doi.org/10.5123/s1679-49742016000100009.
16. Brito AS. Stress and accidents at work: a Pró Sáude study [thesis]. Rio de Janeiro (RJ): Fiocruz; 2007.
17. Brum LM, Azambuja, CR, Rezer, JFP, et al. Quality of life of science teachers in a public school in Rio Grande do Sul. Trab. educ. saúde [online]. 2012 [cited 2015 June 10]; 10(1):125-45. Available from: http://www.scielo.br/ scielo.php?script=sci_arttext&pid=S1981-77462012000100008&lng=en&nrm=iso.
18. Cantley LF, Sherma TB, Slade MD et al. Expert ratings of job demand and job control as predictors of injury and musculoskeletal disorder risk in a manufacturing cohort. Rev.Occup Environ Med. [Internet]. 2015 [cited 2015 August 16]; 0:1-8. Available from: http://oem.bmj.com/content/early/2015/07/10/oemed-2015-102831.long
19. Cardoso HC, Buenor FCC, Mater JC, Alves APR, Jachimst I, Filho IHRV, Hanna MM. Evaluation of sleep quality in medical students. Rev bras de educação médica [Internet]. 2009 [cited 2017 April 20]; 33(3):349 - 355. Available from: http://www.scielo.br/pdf/rbem/v33n3/05.pdf
20. Cavedon NR. Quality of life at work in the area of public security: a diachronic perspective of olfactory perceptions and their implications for the health of civil servants. O&S [Internet]. 2014 [cited 2015 June 9]; 21(68):119-36. Available from: http://www.scielo.br/pdf/osoc/v21n68/a07v21n68.pdf.
21. Unified Workers' Centre. National Secretariat for Labour Relations, Inter-union Department of Statistics and Socioeconomic Studies. Outsourcing and development:

an account that doesn't close: dossier on the impact of outsourcing on workers proposals to guarantee equal rights. São Paulo: Central Única dos Trabalhadores; 2014.

22. Choi KS, Kang SK. Occupational psychiatric disorders in Korea. Korean Med Sci [Internet]. 2010 [cited 2015 Mar 18]; 12(25);S87-S93. Available from: http://dx.doi.org/ 10.3346/jkms.2010.25.S.S87.
23. Chronbach LJ. Coefficient alpha and the internal structure of tests. Psychometrika 1951; 16(3):297-334.
24. Chauvin C, Bouar Le G, Lardjane S. Analysis of occupational injuries in the sea fishing industry according to the type of fishery and the fishing activity. International Maritime Health [Internet]. 2017 [cited 2017 april 14]; 68(1):31- 38. Available from:https://journals.viamedica.pl/international_maritime_health/article/view/49 502
25. Chungkham HS, Michael I, Robert K, et al. Factor structure and longitudinal measurement invariance of the demand control support model: an evidence from the Swedish Longitudinal Occupational Survey of Health (SLOSH). PloS one [Internet]. 2013 [cited 2015 Apr 10]; 8(8):e70541. Available from: http://journals.plos.org/plosone/article?id=10.1371/journal.pone.0070541
26. Corrêa LR. Sustainability in Civil Construction. [monograph]; Federal University of Minas Gerais: Belo Horizonte; 2009.
27. Costa, CSN, Freitas EG, Mendonça LCS, et al. Work ability and quality of life of industrial workers. Ciên & Saúde Coletiva [Internet] 2012 [cited 2015 June 9]; 17(6):1635-42. Available from: http://www.scielosp.org/pdf/csc/v17n6/v17n6a26.pdf.
28. De Queirós AAL, Lima LP. The institutionalisation of the work of community health workers. Trab educ saúde [Internet]. 2012 [cited 2017 April 20];10(2):257-281. Available from: http://www.scielo.br/pdf/tes/v10n2/05.pdf
29. Dos Santos T DeMMD, Inocente NJ. Tadeucci MSR. Occupational Stress in Nurses: Effort-reward risk and super commitment in work. J Nurse UFPE on line [Internet]. 2012 [cited 2017 April 20]; 6(3):488-96 Available from: http://www.revista.ufpe.br/revistaenfermagem/index.php/revista/issue/view/51
30. Dorrian, J. et al. Sleep, stress and compensatory behaviours by Australian nurses and midwives. Rev. Saúde Pública [online]. 2011 [cited 2017 April 20];45(5): 922-930. Available from: http://www.scielo.br/pdf/rsp/v45n5/2538.pdf

31. Dutta MJ. Int J Environ Res Public Health. [Internet] 2017 [cited 2017 April 19]; 29;14(2). pii: E132. Available from: https://www.ncbi.nlm.nih.gov/pubmed/28146056
32. Feder K ,Michaud DS, Keith SE, et al. An assessment of quality of life using the WHOQOL-BREF among participants living in the vicinity of wind turbines. Environ Res. [Internet].2015 [cited 2015 Aug16] Jul 11(142):227-238. Available from: http://www.sciencedirect.com/science/article/pii/S0013935115300189
33. Ferraz RRN, Aquino S. Urinary lithiasis in construction workers as an indicator for health management and improvement in people management. Ciênc. saúde coletiva [Internet]. 2014 Dec [cited 2015 June 9]; 19(12):4759-66. Available from: http://www.scielo.br/scielo.php?script=sci_arttext&pid=S1413- 8123201400120 4759&lng=en.
34. Ferreira LRC, Martino MMF. Sleep pattern and sleepiness of nursing student workers. Rev. esc. enferm. USP [Internet]. 2012 Oct [cited 2015 June 10]; 46(5):1178-83. Available from: http://www.scielo.br/scielo.php?script=sci_arttext& pid=S0080-62342012000500020&lng=en.
35. Ferreira MC, Alves L, Tostes N. Gestão de Qualidade de Vida no Trabalho (QVT) no Serviço Público Federal: O Descompasso entre Problemas e Práticas Gerenciais, Psic.: Teor. e Pesq. [internet]. 2009, [cited 2015 June 9]; 25(3):319-327. Available from: http://www.scielo.br/scielo.php?script=sci_arttext&pid=S0102-3772200 9000300005&lng=pt&nrm=iso.
36. Fischer FM, Moreno CRC, Borges FNS, Louzada FM. Implementation of 12-hour shifts in a Brazilian petrochemical plant: impact on sleep and alertness. Chronobiol Int. 2000;17:521-37.
37. Fossum IN, Bjorvatn B, Waage S, et al. Effects of shift and night work in the offshore petroleum industry: a systematic review. Industrial health [Internet]. 2013 [cited 2015 June 9]; 51(5):530-44. Available from: http://www.ncbi.nlm.nih.gov/pmc/ articles/PMC4202738/.
38. Fujiki N. Sleep problems in occupational health. Journal of UOEH [Intenet]. 2013 [cited 2015 June 9]; 35(Special_Issue):157-62. Occupational Health Physicians and Four Decades of Industrial Safety and Health Law. Language: English-Japanese. Previous Article |Next Article http://doi.org/10.7888/juoeh.35.157

39. Galdino A, Vilma SS, Silvia F. Os Centros de Referência em Saúde do Trabalhador e a notificação de acidentes de trabalho no Brasil [Workers' Health Referral Centres and reporting of work-related injuries in Brazil]. Cad. Saúde Pública [Internet]. 2012 [cited 2015 May 4]; 28(1):145-59. Available from: http://www.scielo.br/pdf/csp/v28n1/15.pdf.
40. Garg R, Cheung JP, Fung BK, Ip WY et al.Epidemiology of occupational hand injury in Hong Kong. Hong Kong Med J. [Internet].2012[cited 2015 August 16]; 18(2):131-6. Available from: http://www.ncbi.nlm.nih.gov/pubmed/22477736
41. Ghisi M, Novara C, Buodo G, et al. Psychological distress and post-traumatic symptoms following occupational accidents. Behav. Sci [Internet]. 2013 Mar [cited 2015 May 4]; 3(4):587-600. Available from: http://www.mdpi.com/2076-328X/3/4/587/htm.
42. Giorgi G, Dubin D, Perez JF. Perceived Organisational Support for Enhancing Welfare at Work: A Regression Tree Model. Frontiers in Psychology [Internet] 2016; [cited 2017 Marc 8] 7:1770. Available from: https://www.ncbi.nlm.nih.gov/pmc/articles/PMC5186753/
43. Golchin M, Attarchi M, Mirzamohammadi E, et al. Assessment of the relationship between Quality of Life and Upper Extremity Impairment Due to Occupational Injuries. Med J Islam Repub Iran [Internet] 2014 [cited 2015 May 4]; 28:15. Available from: http://www.ncbi.nlm.nih.gov/pmc/articles/PMC4153528/.
44. Gralle PBP , Moreno AB, Juvanhol LL, da Fonseca de JM, Melo ECP, Nunes MAA, Toivanen S, Griep RH. Job strain and binge eating among Brazilian workers participating in the ELSA-Brasil study: does BMI matter?J Occup Health. . [Internet] 2017. [cited 2017 Marc 8]Feb4.Available from: https://www.ncbi.nlm.nih.gov/pubmed/
45. Griep RH, Rotenberg L, Landsbergis S, et al. Combined use of work stress models and self-reported health in nursing. Rev. Saúde Publica [Internet]. 2011. [cited 2015 May 4]; 45(1): 145-52. Available from: http://www.previdencia.gov.br/aeps-2013-secao-iv-acidentes-do-trabalho/.
46. Guimarães Mde L R, Hermont AP. Sleep apnea and occupational accidents: Are oral appliances the solution? Indian J Occup Environ Med.[Internet] 2014 [cited 2017 April 16]; 18(2):39-47. Available from: https://www.ncbi.nlm.nih.gov/pmc/articles/PMC4280775/
47. Guimarães LBM, Pessa BSLR, Biguelini PC. Evaluation of the impact of shiftwork

and chronotype on the workers of the imprint and cutting/welding sectors of a flexible packaging manufacturer. Journal work [Internet]. 2012; [cited 2013 Nov 06];41: 1691-1698. Available from: http://iospress.metapress.com/content/812718v837481295/

48. Haghighi S, Yazdi KZ. (2015). Fatigue management in the workplace Psychiatry Journal [Internet]. 2015. . [cited 2015 Aug 15] 24 (1), 12-17. Available from: http://www.ncbi.nlm.nih.gov/pmc/articles/PMC4525425/

49. Harper A, Power M. Steps for checking and cleaning data and computing domain scores for the Whoqol-Bref. WHOQOL Group. 2000 [Aug 2011]. Available from: http://www.ufrgs.br/psiquiatria/psiq/Sintaxe.pdf.

50. Herman J, Kafoa B, Wainiqolo I, et al. Driver sleepiness and risk of motor vehicle crash injuries: A population-based case control study in Fiji (TRIP 12). Injury Int. J. Care Injured [Internet]. 2014 [cited 2015 May 4]; 45(3):586-91. Available from: http://www.sciencedirect.com/science/article/pii/S0020138313002702

51. Itoh H, Yokoyama K, Matsukawa T, Kitamura F. Association between physical activity and sleep-disordered breathing in male Japanese workers: a cross- sectional study. BMC Res Notes. [Internet]. 2017 [cited 2017 April 16]; 9;10(1):37. Available from: https://www.ncbi.nlm.nih.gov/pubmed/28069061

52. Jacobsen HB, Caban-Martinez A, Onyebeke LC, SorensenG, et al. Construction Workers Struggle with a High Prevalence of Mental Distress and this is Associated with Their Pain and Injuries. J Occup Environ Med. [Internet] 2013 [cited 2015 Sep 03]; 55(10): 1197-1204. Available from: http://www.ncbi.nlm.nih.gov/pmc/articles/PMC3795897/

53. Jeon HJ, Kim JH, Kim BN, et al.Sleep quality, posttraumatic stress, depression, and human errors in train drivers: a population-based nationwide study in South Korea. Sleep. [Internet]. 2014 [cited 2015 August 17]; 37(12):1969-75. Available from: http://www.ncbi.nlm.nih.gov/pubmed/25325495

54. Johnson KD, Patel SR, Baur DM, et al. Association of sleep habits with accidents and near misses in United States transportation operators. J Occup Environ Med. [Internet]. 2014 [cited 2015 Mar 14]; 56(5):510-5. Available from: http://www.ncbi.nlm.nih.gov/pmc/articles/PMC4340239/

55. Jurado-Gámez B,aGuglielmi O, Gude F, Buela-Casa G. Workplace Accidents, Absenteeism and Productivity in Patients With Sleep Apnea. Arch Bronconeumol. [Internet] 2015 [cited 2017 April 16]; 51(5):213-218. Available from:

http://www.archbronconeumol.org/en/linkresolver/accidentes-laborales-absentismo-productividad-pacientes/S0300289614002762/

56. Lourenço S, Carnide F, Benavides FG, Lucas R. Psychosocial Work Environment and Musculoskeletal Symptoms among 21-Year-Old Workers: A Population-Based Investigation (2011-2013). Coyne J, ed. PLoS ONE. [Internet] 2015.[cited 2017 Marc 8]10(6):e0130010.Available from: https://www.ncbi.nlm.nih.gov/pmc/articles/PMC4468175
57. Kalte HO, Hosseini AH, Arabzadeh S, et al. Analysis of electrical accidents and the related causes involving citizens who are served by the Western of Tehran. Electronic physician [Internet]. 2014 May [cited 2015 Jun 10]; 6(2):820-6. Available from: http://www.ncbi.nlm.nih.gov/pmc/articles/PMC4324276/pdf/820- 826.pdf.
58. Kanchana S, Sivaprakash P, Joseph S. Studies on Labour Safety in Construction Sites. The Scientific World Journal. [Internet]. 2015 [cited 2017 April 16] 2015:590810. Available from: https://www.ncbi.nlm.nih.gov/pmc/articles/PMC4709774/
59. Kao KY, Spitzmueller C, Cigularov K, Wu H. Linking insomnia to workplace injuries: A moderated mediation model of supervisor safety priority and safety behaviour. J Occup Health Psychol. 2016 [cited 2017 April 16]; 21(1):91-104. Avalialabre from: https://www.ncbi.nlm.nih.gov/pubmed/26011243
60. Khaleghipour S, Mohsen M, Kelishadi R. Circadian type, chronic fatigue, and serum IgM in the shift workers of an industrial organisation. Adv Biomed Res. [Internet]. 2015 [cited 2015 June 14]; 4(61):1-6. Available from: http://www.advbiores.net/ article.asp? issn=2277-9175;year=2015;volume=4;issue=1;spage=61;epage= 61;aulast=Khaleghipour.
61. Kim T, Min H, Jung J. A Mobility-Aware Adaptive Duty Cycling Mechanism for Tracking Objects during Tunnel Excavation. Sensors (Basel). [Internet] 2017 [cited 2017 April 19] 23:17(3). Available from: https://www.ncbi.nlm.nih.gov/pmc/articles/PMC5375721/
62. Lacerda KM, Fernandes RCP, Nobre LCC. Fatal work accidents in Salvador, BA, Brazil: describing an under-reported event and its relationship to urban violence. Rev Bras Saúde Ocup [Internet]. 2014 [cited 2015 June 14]; 39(129):63-74. Available from: http://www.scielo.br/pdf/rbso/v39n129/0303- 7657-rbso-39-129-0063.pdf.
63. Lourenção LG, Moscardini AC, Soler Z.AG. Health and quality of life of resident doctors. Rev Assoc Med Bras [Internet]. 2010 [cited 2015 Mar 14]; 56(1):81-91. Available from: http://www.scielo.br/pdf/ramb/v56n1/21.pdf.

64. Lu IC, Yen Jean MC, Lei SM, et al. BSRS-5 (5-item Brief Symptom Rating Scale) scores affect every aspect of quality of life measured by WHOQOL- BREF in healthy workers. Qual Life Res. [Internet]. 2011 Nov [cited 2015 Mar 14]; 20(9):1469-1475. Available from: http://link.springer.com/article/10.1007/s11136-011-9889-4#page-1

65. Lykouras D, Karkoulias K, Patouchas D, et al. Experience and limited lighting may affect sleepiness of tunnel workers. BMC research notes [Internet]. 2014 [cited 2015 Mar 14]; 7(1):417. Available from: http://www.biomedcentral.com/1756-0500/7/417.

66. Magnago TSBS, Lisboa, MTL, Griep, RH, et al. Psychosocial aspects of work and musculoskeletal disorders in nursing workers. Rev. Latino-Am. Enfermagem [Internet]. 2010 June [cited 2015 June 9]; 18(3):429-35. Available from: http://www.scielo.br/scielo.php?script=sci arttext&pid=S0104-11692010000300019&lng=en.

67. Magnano TSBS, Lisboa, MTL, Griep, RH, et al. Working conditions of nursing professionals: evaluation based on the demand-control model*. Rev. Acta Enfermagem[Internet]. 2010 June [cited 2015 June 23]; 811-17. http://www. scielo. br/pdf/ape/v23n6/15.pdf

68. Magnusson HLL, Chungkham HS, Akerstedt T, et al.The role of sleep disturbances in the longitudinal relationship between psychosocial working conditions, measured by work demands and support, and depression. Rev. Sleep [Internet]. 2014 Dec[cited 2015 Aug 16] 1;37(12):1977-85. Available from: http://www.ncbi.nlm.nih.gov/pubmed/25325503

69. Marcelino P, Cavalcante S. Towards a definition of outsourcing. Cad. CRH [Internet]. 2012 [cited 2015 June 10]; 25(65):331-46. Available from: http://www.scielo.br/ scielo.php?script=sci_arttext&pid=S0103-49792012000200010&lng=en&nrm=iso>.

70. Marconato Rafael Silva, Monteiro Maria Ines. Pain, health perception and sleep: impact on the quality of life of firefighters/rescue professionals. Rev. Latino-Am. Enfermagem [Internet]. 2015; [cited 2017 Apr 17] ; 23(6): 991999. Available from: http://www.scielo.br/scielo.php?script=sci_arttext&pid=S0104-11692015000600991&lng=en.

71. De Martino MMF. Daytime sleep architecture and sleep-wake cycle in nurses working

shifts. Rev. esc. enferm. USP [Internet]. 2009 Mar [cited 2015 June 10]; 43(1):194-9. Available from: http://www.scielo.br/scielo.php?script=sci_arttext &pid=S0080-62342009000100025&lng=en.

72. Martins GA. On reliability and validity. Rev Bras Gest Neg, 2006; 8(20):1-12.
73. Mehrdad R, Seifmanesh S, Chavoshi F, et al. Epidemiology of occupational accidents in Iran based on social security organisation database. Iranian Red Crescent Medical Journal [Internet]. 2014 [cited 2015 Jun 10]; 16(1):e10359. Available from: http://www.ncbi.nlm.nih.gov/pmc/articles/PMC3964417/.
74. Mello Alves MG, Braga VM, Faerstein E, et al. (2015). The demand-control model for job strain: a commentary on different ways to operationalize the exposure variable Demand-control model of job stress: considerations on different ways. Cad. Saúde Pública [Internet] 2015 [cited 2015 June 10]; 31(1):1-5. Available from: http://www.scielo.br/pdf/csp/v31 n1/0102-311X-csp-31 -01 -00208.pdf.
75. Mendes SS, De Martino MMF. Shift work: general health status related to sleep in nursing workers. Rev esc enferm [Internet]. 2012 [cited 2017 April 20];46(6):1471-6. Available from: http://www.scielo.br/pdf/reeusp/v46n6/26.pdf
76. Migration and Health in the Construction Industry: Culturally Centering Voices of Bangladeshi Workers in Singapore.
77. Ministry of Social Security (BR). AEPS 2013 - Section IV - Accidents at Work [Internet]. 2013. [cited 2015 May 4]. Available from: http://www.previdencia.gov.br/aeps-2013-secao-iv-acidentes-do-trabalho.
78. Ministry of Labour and Employment (BR). Rais - Annual Social Information Report [Internet]. 2013 [cited 2015 June 10]; [about 1 screen]. Available from: http://portal.mte.gov.br/portal-mte/rais/.
79. Mohebbi I, Shateri K , Seyed MM. The Relationship between working schedule patterns and the markers of metabolic syndrome: comparison of shift workers with day workers. International Journal of Occupational Medicine and Environmental Health [Internet]. 2012 [cited 2013 Nov 06];25(4):1. Available from: www.ncbi.nlm.nih.gov/pubmed/23022229
80. Moradinazar M, Kurd N, Farhadi R, et al. Epidemiology of Work-Related Injuries Among Construction Workers of Ilam (Western Iran) During 2006-2009. Iran Red Crescent Med J. [Internet] 2013 [cited 2015 June 9]; 15(10):e8011. Available from: http://www.ncbi.nlm.nih.gov/pmc/articles/PMC3950784/.
81. Ogata A, Simurro S. Practical Guide to Quality of Life: how to plan and manage the

best programme for your company. Rio de Janeiro: Elsevier; 2009.

82. Oliveira RC, Santos JN, Rabelo ATV, et al. The impact of noise exposure on workers in Mobile Support Units. CODAS [Internet]. 2015 June [cited 2015 August 16]; 27 (3): 215-222. Available from: http://www.scielo.br/scielo.php?script=sci_arttext&pid=S2317-17822015000300215&lng=en.

83. Padilha, V. Qualidade de vida no trabalho num cenário de precariousização: a panacea delirante [Quality of work life in a setting of precariousness: a delusional panacea]. Trab. educ. saúde [Internet]. 2009 [cited 2015 June 9]; 7(3):549-63. Available from: http://www.scielo.br/scielo.php?script=sci_serial&pid=1981-7746&nrm=iso&lng=en,

84. Pagano M, Gauvreau K. Principles of Biostatistics. São Paulo: Ed. Thomson; 2004.

85. Paterson JL, Clarkson L, Rainbird S, et al. Occupational fatigue and other health and safety issues for young Australian workers: an exploratory mixed methods study. J. Stage [Internet]. 2015 [cited 2015 June 9]; 53(3):293-9. Available from from: https://www.jstage.jst.go.jp/article/indhealth/advpub/0/advpub_2014-0257/_article.

86. Penteado RZ, Pereira IMTB. Quality of life and vocal health of teachers. Rev. Saúde Pública [Internet]. 2007 [cited 2015 June 10]; 41(2):236-43. Available from: http://www.scielo.br/scielo.php?script=sci_arttext&pid=S0034- 89102007000200010&lng=en.

87. Piotrowski PJ , Robak S , Polewaczyk MM , Raczkowski R. [Offshore substation workers' exposure to harmful factors - Actions minimising risk of hazards]. Med Pr. [Internet] 2016 [cited 2017 April 16] ; 67(1):51-72. Available from: https://www.ncbi.nlm.nih.gov/pubmed/27044719

88. Prakash S, Khapre P, Laha SK, et al. Study to assess the level of stress and identification of significant stressors among the railway engine pilots.Indian J Occup Environ Med. [Internet]. 2011 [cited 2015 Aug 17] 15(3):113- 9.Avaialable from: http://www.ncbi.nlm.nih.gov/pubmed/22412289.

89. Prestes MRD, Feitosa MAG, Sampaio ALL, et al. Can auditory neuropathy spectrum disorder contribute to work accidents? a clinical investigation report. Rev. bras. saúde ocup. [Internet]. 2012 [cited 2015 June 10]; 37(125):181-8. Available from: http://www.scielo.br/scielo.php?pid=S0303-76572012000100021&script=sci_arttext.

90. Raja JD, Kumar BS, Tupil KA, et al. Stress, anxiety, and depression among call handlers employed in international call centres in the national capital region of Delhi. Indian J Public Health [Internet]. 2015 [cited 2015 June 10]; 59(2):95- 101. Available from: http://www.ijph.in/citation.asp?issn=0019-557X;year=2015;volume=59;issue=2; spage=95;epage=101;aulast=Jeyapal;aid=IndianJPublicHealth_2015_59_2_95_157508.
91. Rameezdeen R, Elmualim A The Impact of Heat Waves on Occurrence and Severity of Construction Accidents Int. J. Environ. Res. Public Health [Internet] 2017 [cited 2017 April 14] 14(1), 70. Available from: https://www.ncbi.nlm.nih.gov/pmc/articles/PMC5295321/
92. Rios KA, Barbosa DA, Belasco AGS. Assessment of quality of life and depression in nursing technicians and assistants. Rev. Latino-Am. Enfermagem [Internet]. 2010 June [cited 2015 June 10]; 18(3):413-20. Available from: http://www.scielo.br/scielo. php?script=sci_arttext&pid=S0104-11692010000300017&lng=en.
93. Rocha KB, Muntaner C, Solar O, et al. Clase social, factores de riesgo psicossocial en el trabajo y su asociación con la salud autopercibida y mental en Chile. Cad. Saúde Pública Internet]. 2014 Oct [cited 2015 June 9]; 30(10):2219-34. Available from: http://www.scielo.br/scielo.php?script=sci_arttext&pid=S0102-311X201400 1002219&lng=en.
94. Roenneberg T, Kuehnle T, Pramstaller PP, et al. A marker for the end of adolescence. Curr Biol [Internet]. 2004 [cited 2015 June 11]; 14(24):1038- R1039. Available from: http://www.sciencedirect.com/science/article/pii/ S0960982204009285.
95. Rusli BN, Edimansyah BA, Naing L. Working conditions, self-perceived stress, anxiety, depression and quality of life: a structural equation modelling approach. RevBMC Public Health[Intertnet].2008 [cited 2015 Aug 16]; 6(8):48.Available from: http://www.ncbi.nlm.nih.gov/pubmed/18254966
96. Santos LC, Goulart Júnior E, Canêo LC, et al. Psychology and the profession: professional neurosis and the role of the organisational psychologist in dealing with the issue. Psicol cienc prof [Internet]. 2010. [cited 2015 June 9]; 30(2) :248-61. Available from: http://www.scielo.br/scielo.php?pid=S1414-98932010000200003&script=sci_arttext.
97. SAS/STAT®. User's Guide, Version 9.2. Cary, NC, USA: SAS Institute Inc; 2008.

98. Schioler L, Soderberg M, Rosengren A, et al. Psychosocial work environment and risk of ischemic stroke and coronary heart disease: a prospective longitudinal study of 75 236 construction workers. Scand J Work Environ Health [Internet]. 2015 [cited 2015 June 9]; 41(3):280-7. Available from: http://www.sjweh.fi/order_document.php.

99. Serkalem S, Haimanot GM, Ansha, NA. Determinants of Occupational Injury in Kombolcha Textile Factory, North-East Ethiopia. J. Occup. Environ. Med [Internet]. 2014 [cited 2015 June 9]; 5(2): 327-84. Available from: http://www.theijoem.com/ijoem/index.php/ijoem/article/view/327/467.

100. Silva, CA, Ferreira MC. Dimensions and indicators of quality of life and well-being at work. Psychology: Theory and Research [Internet] 2013 [cited 2015 May 5] 29(3):331-9. Available from: http://www.scielo.br/pdf/ptp/v29n3/v29n3a11.pdf.

101. Simões ALB, Martino MMF. Circadian variability of oral, tympanic and axillary temperature in hospitalised adults. Rev esc enferm [Internet]. 2007 [cited 2013 Nov 6]; 41(3):485-91. Available from: http://www.scielo.br/pdf/reeusp/v41n3/20.pdf.

102. Socias, CM, Menéndez CKC, Collins, JW, et al. Occupational Ladder Fall Injuries- United States-2011. Morbidity and mortality weekly report MMWR [Internet]. 2014 April 25 [cited 2015 June 9] 63(16) 343. Available from:www.cdc.gov/mmwr/ pdf/wk/mm6316.pdf.

103. Sotelo-Suárez NR, Quiroz-Arcentáles JL, Quiroz-Arcentáles CP, et al. Condiciones de salud y trabajo de las mujeres en la economía informal Bogotá 2007. Rev Salud Pública [Internet]. 2012 [cited 2015 June 9]; 14(1):32-42. Available from: http://www.scielo.org.co/pdf/rsap/v14s1/v14s1a04.pdf.

104. Soh M, Zarola A, Palaiou K, Furnham A. Work-related well-being. Health psychology open. [Internet] 2016 [cited 2017 Mar 9];3(1):2055102916628380.Available from: https://www.ncbi.nlm.nih.gov/pmc/articles/PMC5193259

105. Sridhar GR, Sanjana NS. Sleep, circadian dysrhythmia, obesity and diabetes World J Diabetes. [Internet] 2016 [cited 2017 April 17]; 15;7(19):515- 522. Available from: https://www.ncbi.nlm.nih.gov/pubmed/27895820

106. Suárez SFA, Carvajal PGI, Catalá AJ. Occupational safety and health in construction: a review of applications and trends. Ind Health. [Internet] 2017 [cited April 14] Feb 7. Available from:

https://www.jstage.jst.go.jp/article/indhealth/advpub/0/advpub 2016-0108/ pdf

107. Suri S, Das R Occupational health profile of workers employed in the manufacturing sector of India. Natl Med J India. [Internet] 2016 S[cited April 16] 29(5):277-281 .Available from: https://www.ncbi.nlm.nih.gov/pubmed/28098082

108. Tabeleão VP, Tomasi E, Neves SF. Quality of life and professional burnout among public high school and elementary school teachers in southern Brazil. Cad. Saúde Pública [Internet]. 2011 [cited 2017 Mar 08] ; Dec 27(12):2401-2408.Available from: http://www.scielo.br/scielo.php?script=sci arttext&pid=S0102-311X2011001200011&

109. Thielen K1, Nygaard E, Andersen I, Diderichsen F.Employment consequences of depressive symptoms and work demands individually and combined.Eur J Public Health. [Internet] 2014 cited 2017 Mar 08] Feb;24(1):34-9. Available from:https://academic.oup.com/eurpub/article-lookup

110. Tomei G., Capozzella A, Rosati MV, et al. Stress e infortuni sul lavoro. Clin Ter [Internet]. 2015 [cited 2015 June 9]; 166(1):e7-22. Available from: http://www.seu-roma.it/riviste/clinica_ terapeutica/open_access/articoli/e49f83f395b2bc43f42b 12cc6e2614b6.pdf.

111. Ulhôa M, Moreno CRC. Psychosocial Factors at Work and Cortisol: A Brief Review Revista InterfacHES [Internet]. 2009 [cited 2015 June 9]; 4(3). Available from: http://www.revistas.sp.senac.br/index.php/ITF/article/view/49.

112. Vegso S, Cantley L, Slade M, et al. Extended work hours and risk of acute occupational injury: A case-crossover study of workers in manufacturing. Am J Ind Med [Internet]. 2007 Aug [cited 2015 June 11]; 50(8):597-603. Available from: http://onlinelibrary.wiley.com/doi/10.1002/ajim.20486/abstract doi:10.1002/ajim.20486

113. Vilela RAG, Almeida IM, Mendes RW. From surveillance to prevention of work accidents: contribution of activity ergonomics. Rev Cien & Saúde Coletiva [Internet]. 2012 [cited 2015 June 4]; 17(10). Available from:www.scielosp.org/ pdf/csc/v17n10/29.pdf.

114. Virtanen M, Nyberg ST, Batty GD, et al. Perceived job insecurity as a risk factor for incident coronary heart disease: systematic review and meta-analysis. BMJ [Internet]. 2013 [cited 2013 Aug 8]; 347:f4746. Available from: http://www.ncbi.nlm.nih.gov/ pmc/articles/PMC3738256/.

115. Yi W, Chan A. Health Profile of Construction Workers in Hong Kong.

Tchounwou PB, ed. International Journal of Environmental Research and Public Health. [Internet] 2016 [cited 2017 April 14] 13(12):1232. Available from: https://www.ncbi.nlm.nih.gov/pmc/articles/PMC5201373/

116. Wagstaff AS, Sigstad Lie JA. Shift and night work and long working hours - a systematic review of safety implications. Scand J Work Environ Health [Internet]. 2011 [cited 2014 Aug 8]; 37(3):173-185 Available from: http://www.ncbi.nlm.nih.gov/ pubmed/21290083.

ANNEXES

ANNEX A - INFORMED CONSENT FORM

We invite you to take part in the research project "Construction workers, chronotype and the prevalence of accidents", which will be carried out by a doctoral nurse from the postgraduate nursing programme at the Federal University of the State of São Paulo - Unifesp.

This project aims to understand the prevalence of accidents among construction workers: repercussions on quality of life and chronotype.

Interviews will be carried out to collect the data. This does not entail any risks or discomfort, but we hope it will bring you benefits related to helping you gain a greater understanding of what can influence the occurrence of accidents at work among workers in outsourced construction companies.

You will be guaranteed that your name and any other data that identifies you will be kept confidential and that you will be free to withdraw from participating in the research at any time, without this causing you any harm.

After reading this consent form and agreeing to take part in the research, please sign it. Any additional information or clarification regarding the research can be obtained from the researcher in charge, master's degree nurse Roberta Zaninelli do Nascimento Zarpelão (Nurse COREN/SP 0014039)."

E-mail: rzn.zarpelao@unifesp.br

Me,..

I hereby declare my consent to participate as a subject in the study: "The prevalence of accidents among construction workers: repercussions on quality of life and chronotype" I also declare that I am aware of its objectives and method, as well as my right to withdraw at any time, without any penalty and/or prejudice to the care I receive. I authorise the use of a tape recorder to record the interview and a photographic record if necessary.

Name: ____

Signature: ____

RG: 6.145859-0 SSP PR..

Signature of the researcher responsible; ____ .

Cubatão, of 2013.

UNIVERSIDADE FEDERAL DE
SÃO PAULO - UNIFESP/
HOSPITAL SÃO PAULO

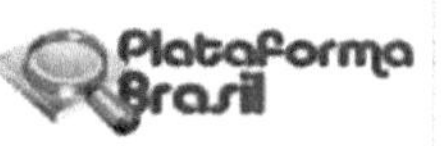

Continuação do Parecer: 319.253

Situação do Parecer:

Aprovado

Necessita Apreciação da CONEP:

Não

Considerações Finais a critério do CEP:

O colegiado acata o parecer do relator.

SAO PAULO, 28 de Junho de 2013

Assinador por:
José Osmar Medina Pestana
(Coordenador)

Endereço: Rua Botucatu, 572 1º Andar Conj. 14
Bairro: VILA CLEMENTINO **CEP:** 04.023-061
UF: SP **Município:** SAO PAULO
Telefone: (11)5539-7162 **Fax:** (11)5571-1062 **E-mail:** cepunifesp@unifesp.br

ANNEX B

CONTROL DEMAND QUESTIONNAIRE

	QUESTIONÁRIO DEMANDA CONTROLE			
SEXO:	IDADE:			
TEMPO DE PROFISSÃO	FUNÇÃO			
PARTE DO CORPO ATINGIDA:				
A) COM QUE FREQUENCIA VOCÊ TEM QUE FAZER SUAS TAREFAS DE TRABALHO COM MUITA RAPIDEZ?	3 RARAMENTE	1 FREQUENTEMENTE	2 ÀS VEZES	4 NUNCA
B) COM QUE FREQUENCIA VOCÊ TEM QUE TRABALHAR INTENSAMENTE (ISTO É, PRODUZIR MUITO EM POUCO TEMPO?	RARAMENTE	FREQUENTEMENTE	ÀS VEZES	NUNCA
C) SEU TRABALHO EXIGE DEMAIS DE VOCÊ?	RARAMENTE	FREQUENTEMENTE	ÀS VEZES	NUNCA
D) VOCÊ TEM TEMPO PARA CUMPRIR TODAS AS TAREFAS DO SEU TRABALHO?	RARAMENTE	FREQUENTEMENTE	ÀS VEZES	NUNCA
E) O SEU TRABALHO COSTUMA APRESENTAR EXIGÊNCIAS CONTRADITÓRIAS OU DISCORDANTES?	RARAMENTE	FREQUENTEMENTE	ÀS VEZES	NUNCA
F) VOCÊ TEM POSSIBILIDADE DE APRESENTAR COISAS NOVAS EM SEU TRABALHO?	RARAMENTE	FREQUENTEMENTE	ÀS VEZES	NUNCA
G) SEU TRABALHO EXIGE MUITA HABILIDADE OU CONHECIMENTOS ESPECIALIZADOS?	RARAMENTE	FREQUENTEMENTE	ÀS VEZES	NUNCA
H) SEU TRABALHO EXIGE QUE VC TOME INICIATIVAS?	RARAMENTE	FREQUENTEMENTE	ÀS VEZES	NUNCA
I) NO SEU TRABALHO VC TEM COMO REPETIR MUITAS VEZES AS MESMAS TAREFAS?	RARAMENTE	FREQUENTEMENTE	ÀS VEZES	NUNCA
J) VOCÊ PODE ESCOLHER **COMO** FAZER O SEU TRABALHO?	RARAMENTE	FREQUENTEMENTE	ÀS VEZES	NUNCA
K) VOCÊ PODE ESCOLHER **O QUE FAZER** O SEU TRABALHO?	RARAMENTE	FREQUENTEMENTE	ÀS VEZES	NUNCA
L) EXISTE UM AMBIENTE CALMO E AGRADÁVEL EM SEU TRABALHO?	4 CONCORDO TOTAL	3 CONCORDO+QUE DISCORDO	2 DISCORDO+ CONCORDO	1 DISCORDO TOTALMENTE
M) NO TRABALHO NOS RELACIONAMOS BEM UNS COM OS OUTROS?	CONCORDO TOTAL	CONCORDO+QUE DISCORDO	DISCORDO+ CONCORDO	DISCORDO TOTALMENTE
N) EU POSSO CONTAR COM O APOIO DOS MEUS COLEGAS DE TRABALHO?	CONCORDO TOTAL	CONCORDO+QUE DISCORDO	DISCORDO+ CONCORDO	DISCORDO TOTALMENTE
O) SE EU NÃO ESTIVER NUM BOM DIA MEUS COLEGAS COMPREENDEM?	CONCORDO TOTAL	CONCORDO+QUE DISCORDO	DISCORDO+ CONCORDO	DISCORDO TOTALMENTE
P) NO TRABALHO EU ME RELACIONO BEM COM OS COLEGAS?	CONCORDO TOTAL	CONCORDO+QUE DISCORDO	DISCORDO+ CONCORDO	DISCORDO TOTALMENTE
Q) EU GOSTO DE TRABALHAR COM MEUS COLEGAS?	CONCORDO TOTAL	CONCORDO+QUE DISCORDO	DISCORDO+ CONCORDO	DISCORDO TOTALMENTE

ANNEX C

QUALITY OF LIFE QUESTIONNAIRE - WHOQOL-bref

Instructions

This questionnaire is about how you feel about your quality of life, health and other areas of your life. **Please answer all the questions.** If you are not sure which answer to give to a question, please choose from the alternatives the one that seems most appropriate to you. This can often be your first choice. Please bear in mind your values, aspirations, pleasures and concerns. We are asking you how you feel about your life, with reference to the **last two weeks.**

Please read each question, see what you think and circle the number that you think is the best answer.

		Very bad	Bad	Neither bad nor good	Good	Very good
1	How would you rate your quality of life?	1	2	3	4	5

		Very satisfied	Dissatisfied	Not happy Nor dissatisfied	Satisfied	Very satisfied
2	How satisfied are you with your health?	1	2	3	4	5

The following questions are about how you've been feeling things over the last few weeks.

		Nothing	Very little	More or less	Quite a lot	Extreme mind
3	To what extent do you think your (physical) pain prevents you from doing what you need to do?	1	2	3	4	5
4	0 how much medical treatment do you need to go about your daily life?	1	2	3	4	5
5	0 how much do you enjoy your life?	1	2	3	4	5
6	How meaningful do you think your life is?	1	2	3	4	5
7	0 how much you can your self focus?	1	2	3	4	5
8	How safe do you feel in your daily life?	1	2	3	4	5
9	How healthy is your physical environment (climate, noise, pollution, attractions)?	1	2	3	4	5

The following questions ask how fully you have felt or are able to do certain things in the past two weeks.

		Nothing	Very little	Medium	A lot	Complete the mind
10	Do you have enough energy for your day-to-day life?	1	2	3	4	5
11	Are you able to accept your physical appearance?	1	2	3	4	5
12	Do you have enough money to satisfy their needs?	1	2	3	4	5
13	How available is the information that need in your day-to-day life?	1	2	3	4	5
14	To what extent do you have leisure opportunities?	1	2	3	4	5

The following questions ask how good or satisfied you have felt about various aspects of your life in the last two weeks?

		Very bad	Bad	Not bad Not good	Good	Very good
15	How well can you to yourself getting around?	1	2	3	4	5
16	How satisfied are you with your sleep?	1	2	3	4	5
17	How satisfied are you with your ability to carry out your day-to-day activities?	1	2	3	4	5
18	How satisfied are you with your ability to do the job?	1	2	3	4	5
19	How satisfied are you with yourself?	1	2	3	4	5
20	How satisfied you are with your personal relationships (friends , relatives, acquaintanc es, colleagues)?	1	2	3	4	5
21	How satisfied are you with your sex life?	1	2	3	4	5
22	How satisfied are you with the support you receive from your friends?	1	2	3	4	5
23	How satisfied are you with the conditions where you live?	1	2	3	4	5

24	How satisfied are you with your access to health services?	1	2	3	4	5
25	How satisfied are you with your means of transport?	1	2	3	4	5

The following questions refer to how often you have felt or experienced certain things in the last two weeks.

		Never	Sometimes	Often	Very frequent	Always
26	With which frequency you have negative feelings such as low mood, despair, anxiety, depression?	1	2	3	4	5

Did anyone help you fill in this questionnaire?

How long did it take you to fill in this questionnaire?

Do you have any comments on the questionnaire?

THANKS FOR YOUR CO-OPERATION

ANNEX D

MUNICH CHRONOTYPE QUESTIONNAIRE (MCQT)

Questionário de Cronótipo de Munique (QCTM)

Data: ______________

Idade: _____ Feminino☐ Masculino☐ Altura: _____ cm Peso: ____ kg

Quantos dias trabalho por semana? 0☐ 1☐ 2☐ 3☐ 4☐ 5☐ 6☐ 7☐

Tem trabalhado em algum tipo de trabalho por turnos nos últimos 3 meses? sim ☐ não☐

É um fumador? sim ☐ não ☐

Se "sim": Quantos cigarros, em média, fuma por dia? ______________

Por favor, complete <u>todas as</u> secções, independentemente de trabalhar numa base regular ou não. Use a escala das 24 horas, por exemplo, 23:00 em vez de 11:00!!!!

① ② ③ ④ ⑤ ⑥

Nos dias de trabalho (incluindo a noite anterior ao primeiro dia de trabalho)

... vou para a cama às ________ horas **(veja a figura 1)**

... às ________ horas, decido ir dormir **(veja a figura 3)**

... necessito de ________ minutos para adormecer **(veja a figura 4)**

... acordo às ________ horas **(veja a figura 5)**

sem despertador ☐ com despertador ☐

... passados ________ minutos acordo **(veja a figura 6)**

Em média,

quanto tempo, anda na rua exposto à luz do dia (sem um chapéu na cabeça)? ____h ____min

Fora dos dias de trabalho (incluindo a noite anterior ao primeiro dia de descanso ou lazer)

... vou para a cama às ________ horas **(veja a figura 1)**

... às ________ horas, decido ir dormir **(veja a figura 3)**

... necessito de ________ minutos para adormecer **(veja a figura 4)**

... acordo às ________ horas **(veja a figura 5)**

sem despertador ☐ com despertador ☐

... passados ________ minutos acordo **(veja a figura 6)**

Em média,

quanto tempo, anda na rua exposto à luz do dia (sem um chapéu na cabeça)? ____h ____min

Número de Código (do not fill out) ______________________________

MCTQ, 1.2(E)

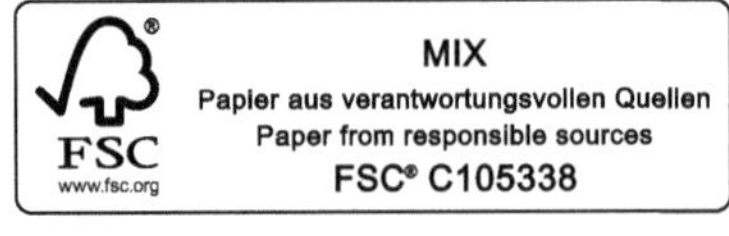

Printed by Books on Demand GmbH, Norderstedt / Germany